YOGA TWISTS and TURNS

YOGA TWISTS and TURNS

50 Sequences to Take Your Practice to the Next Level

Emma Silverman

Photographs by Leslie D. Davis
Modeled by Kelsie Besaw

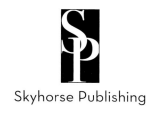

Skyhorse Publishing

Skyhorse Publishing books may be purchased in bulk at special discounts for sales promotion, corporate gifts, fund-raising, or educational purposes. Special editions can also be created to specifications. For details, contact the Special Sales Department, Skyhorse Publishing, 307 West 36th Street, 11th Floor, New York, NY 10018 or info@skyhorsepublishing.com.

Skyhorse® and Skyhorse Publishing® are registered trademarks of Skyhorse Publishing, Inc.®, a Delaware corporation.

www.skyhorsepublishing.com

10 9 8 7 6 5 4 3 2 1

Library of Congress Cataloging-in-Publication Data is available on file.

Cover design by Jane Sheppard

Print ISBN: 978-1-5107-0312-4
Ebook ISBN: 978-1-5107-0313-1

Printed in China

To YY, unreasonably

Table of Contents

Introduction

This is the book you were wondering if you were ready for—and I'm here to tell you that, yes, you are ready. You've been doing yoga consistently for a few months, or on and off for a number of years. Maybe you've been practicing for even longer. There are poses that you see other students doing and you wonder: CAN MY BODY DO THAT?

In my first book, THE JOY OF YOGA, I created a series of sequences for everyday needs and experiences. Belly ache? Check. Waiting for the water to boil? Sure thing. In this book, I'm kicking it up a notch. In YOGA TWISTS AND TURNS, the sequences lead to specific intermediate and advanced poses regularly taught in yoga classes that may seem out of reach. Worried about trying to "Flip Your Dog" in a room filled with yogis? First flip to page 72 for "Wild Thing" in the Heart Openers chapter, where I'll tell you an exact series of postures that will warm up your body to safely move into the ASANA. Curious about how to practice some of your favorite studio poses at home, but without throwing your back out? Here are sequences that will teach you how to prep for a pose in your living room, on the beach, or wherever it is you get your yoga on.

The book is divided thematically into five chapters with ten unique challenge poses per chapter. The final sequence of the book is a restorative series of poses that perfectly top off any sequence (SAVASANA, of course, included). If you're looking to try out a particular pose, turn to that page and follow the sequence. Afterward, either flow with the cooldown of your choosing or follow the restorative sequence. If you're looking for a mood more than a pose, then head to the chapter that sounds yummiest and roll out your mat.

As with any intense physical practice, check in with your yoga teacher or physician before trying these poses. This book teaches the warm-ups for the yoga poses, but does not go into their correct alignment (there are a ton of great books out there that do that!). It's best that you see these poses in the studio first before refining and mastering them at home. If you see a pose in this book you've never seen in the studio (but looks pretty sweet), ask about it! We yoga teachers love to talk about yoga (*A LOT*).

The practice of yoga teaches us to live in the moment and to be present throughout all of life's twists and turns. Your yoga practice is ready to experience *MORE* stretch, *MORE* strength, and *MORE* poses. That way you'll be ready for anything—on or off the mat. So, what are you waiting for? Dive into *YOGA TWISTS AND TURNS*, starting now!

Sun Salutations

While the origins of the Sun Salutations (*Surya Namaskar*) might be debatable, the ubiquity of this series in the modern-day yoga studio is definite. The sequence of poses that are shown here are practiced in a style of yoga called *Ashtanga*. That said, numerous variations exist and have similar health and wellness benefits.

There are a couple of reasons that these two sequences are set aside from the rest. Primarily, I will sometimes refer to the Sun Salutations as a step in a larger sequence without writing out each individual pose within the Sun Salutations. That way, you can flip back to this page as a reference while you're still learning the Sun Salutations and later you can move through the flow without needing to check. In addition, this fun and vibrant sequence is usually practiced as a warm-up to other yoga poses, but can be a great stand-alone sequence if you only have a few minutes to spare and could use a yoga wake-up call.

Feel free to add in a Sun Salutations (or twelve) to any sequence in this book. You'll feel more energized, fired up, and radiant—just like the sun!

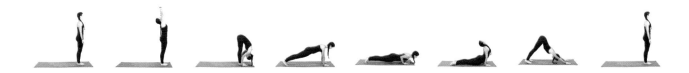

Sun Salutations A

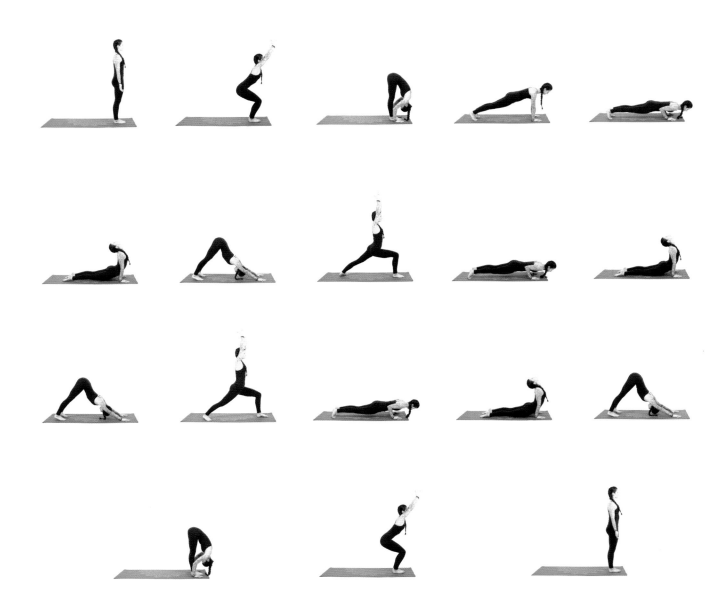

Sun Salutations B

Ground Down

Standing Poses

Pyramid Pose (Parsvottanasana)

The more literal translation of this pose's name (from Sanskrit to English) is Intense Side Stretch Pose. They aren't kidding. This posture provides an amazing hamstring stretch while simultaneously lengthening the spine and allowing the neck to release. Although there are many modifications for this posture available to all levels of yoga students, the full version of this pose has the hands pressed together behind the back in reverse prayer position (ANJALI MUDRA). This sequence will help prep your wrists and legs for an Intense Stretch!

1. *TADASANA* (Mountain Pose)
2. *SURYA NAMASKAR A* (Sun Salutation A—see page 1). Repeat 6 times.
3. *UTKATASANA* (Chair Pose)
4. *PARIVRTTA UTKATASANA* (Revolved Chair Pose). Repeat on other side.
5. *UTTANASANA* (Standing Forward Fold). Hold for 2–3 minutes.
6. *URDHVA HASTASANA* (Upward Hands Pose). Note: Reach one hand higher and then the other, alternating side stretches.
7. *TRIKONASANA* (Triangle Pose). Repeat on other side.
8. *PRASARITA PADOTTANASANA* (Standing Wide-Legged Forward Fold)
9. *BADDHA KONASANA* (Bound Angle Pose)
10. *GOMUKHASANA* (Cow Face Pose). Repeat other side.
11. *PASCHIMOTTANASANA* (Seated Forward Fold)
12. *PARSVOTTANASANA* (Pyramid Pose). Repeat on other side.

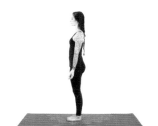

1 Tadasana

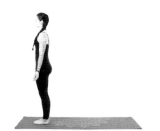

2 Sun Salutation A—
    see page 1

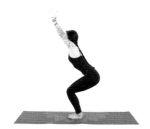

3 Utkatasana

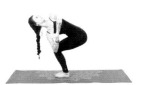

4 Parivrtta
    Utkatasana

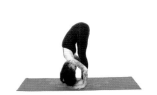

5 Uttanasana

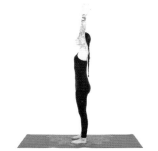

6 Urdhva
    Hastasana

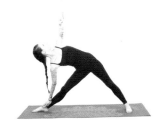

7 Trikonasana

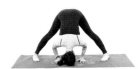

8 Prasarita
    Padottanasana

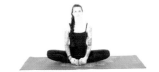

9 Baddha Konasana

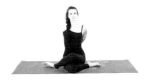

10 Gomukhasana

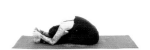

11 Paschimottanasana

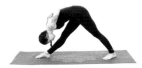

12 Parsvottanasana

Revolved Triangle Pose (Parivrtta Trikonasana)

In my classes, I like to say that poses should feel at least one of two ways: either good or good for you. Let's just say that, in my experience, Revolved Triangle Pose feels really, really good for me. While you're getting the hang of this abdominal twist, shoulder opener, and leg strengthener, I recommend using a block for the lower hand and keeping the top hand on the lower back.

1. *Baddha Konasana* (Bound Angle Pose)
2. *Ardha Matsyendrasana* (Half Seated Twist Pose). Repeat on other side.
3. *Uttanasana* (Standing Forward Fold). Hold for 2-3 minutes.
4. *Tadasana* (Mountain Pose)
5. *Surya Namaskar A* (Sun Salutation A—see page 1). Repeat 5 times.
6. *Utkatasana* (Chair Pose)
7. *Parivrtta Utkatasana* (Revolved Chair Pose). Repeat on other side.
8. *Virabhadrasana II* (Warrior II)
9. *Baddha Virabhadrasana* (Humble Warrior Pose)

Continued on page 8.

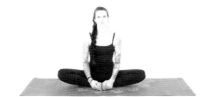

1 Baddha Konasana

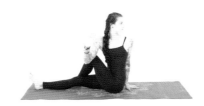

2 Ardha Matsyendrasana

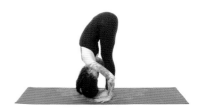

3 Uttanasana

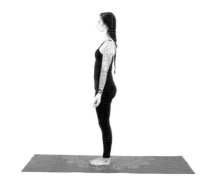

4 Tadasana

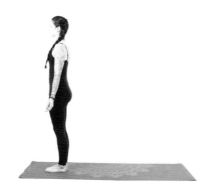

5 Sun Salutation A—
see page 1

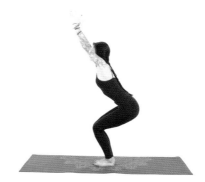

6 Utkatasana

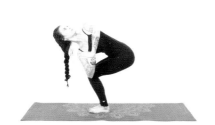

7 Parivrtta Utkatasana

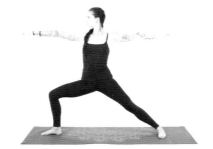

8 Virabhadrasana II

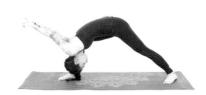

9 Baddha Virabhadrasana

10. *Viparita Virabhadrasana* (Peaceful Warrior Pose)

11. *Utthita Parsvakonasana* (Extended Side Angle Pose)

12. *Trikonasana* (Triangle Pose)

13. *Prasarita Padottanasana* (Standing Wide-Legged Forward Fold), with *Gomukhasana* (Cow Face Pose) bind in the arms

14. *Parsvottanasana* (Pyramid Pose)

15. *Parivrtta Trikonasana* (Revolved Triangle Pose)

16. *Vinyasa* to repeat steps 6 through 15 on other side, alternating which arm is on top in step 13.

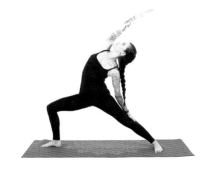

10 Viparita Virabhadrasana

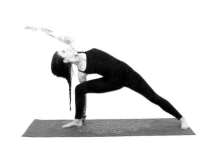

11 Utthita Parsvakonasana

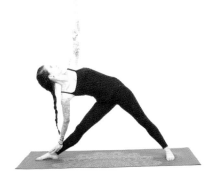

12 Trikonasana

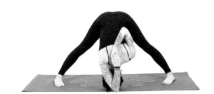

13 Prasarita Padottanasana
with Gomukhasana

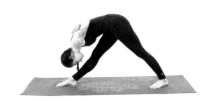

14 Parsvottanasana

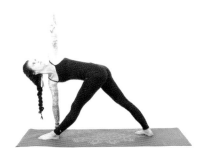

15 Parivrtta Trikonasana

Warrior III Pose (*Virabhadrasana III*)

Warrior III has a number of variations accessible to anyone, including a variation for the Chair Yoga class I teach (in that class, we hold onto a chair with both hands). The more traditional Warrior III extends both arms alongside the ears while the entire torso and hovering leg remain parallel to the earth. This requires great leg, abdominal, and full back strength. The game changer for me in this pose was to think about pressing the thigh bone of the standing leg backward while simultaneously shifting weight onto the heel of my foot. That, and learning to enjoy core work (I can't promise the second one will come as easily).

1. Begin by lying on belly
2. Sphinx Pose
3. *Bhujangasana* (Cobra Pose)
4. *Makrasana* (Crocodile Pose)
5. *Balasana* (Child's Pose)
6. Cat/Cow in Table Top
7. *Navasana* (Boat Pose). Repeat twice more.
8. *Adho Mukha Svanasana* (Downward Facing Dog Pose). Note: Take some time here to pedal the heels in place.

Continued on page 12.

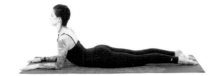

2   Sphinx

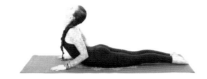

3   Bhujangasana

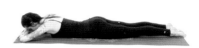

4   Makrasana

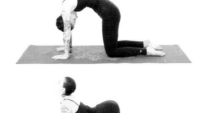

5   Balasana

6   Cat/Cow in Table Top

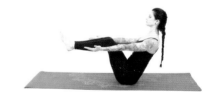

7   Navasana

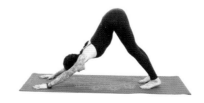

8   Adho Mukha Svanasana

9. *Uttanasana* (Standing Forward Fold)

10. *Utkatasana* (Chair Pose)

11. *Virabhadrasana I* (Warrior I Pose)

12. *Virabhadrasana II* (Warrior II Pose)

13. *Trikonasana* (Triangle Pose)

14. *Alanasana* (High Lunge Pose)

15. *Virabhadrasana III* (Warrior III Pose)

16. Repeat steps 10 through 15 on other side.

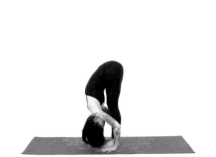

9 Uttanasana

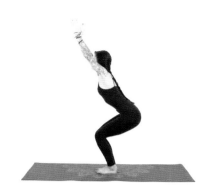

10 Utkatasana

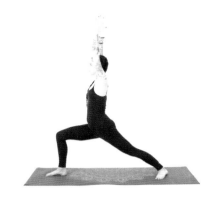

11 Virabhadrasana I

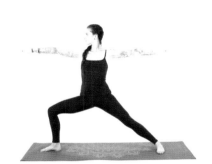

12 Virabhadrasana II

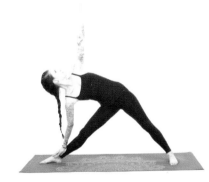

13 Trikonasana

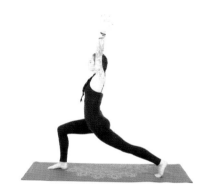

14 Alanasana

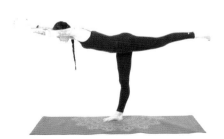

15 Virabhadrasana III

Balancing Half Moon Pose (Ardha Chandrasana)

One of my favorite ways to do this pose is to lean the entire back of my body into a wall. In addition to feeling like I could be there all day (and even make a few phone calls) it helps remind me of the proper alignment of the pose: shoulders, ribs, and hips all in the same plane.

1. *Paschimottanasana* (Seated Forward Fold)
2. *Supta Padangusthasana* (Reclined Big Toe Pose)
3. *Supta Trivikramasana* (Reclined Vishnu Pose)
4. *Ananda Balasana* (Happy Baby Pose)
5. Repeat step 2 through 4 on other side.
6. *Supta Baddha Konasana* (Reclined Bound Angle Pose)
7. *Adho Mukha Svanasana* (Downward Facing Dog Pose)

Continued on page 16.

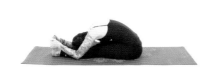

1 Paschimottanasana

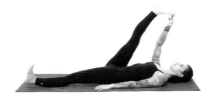

2 Supta Padangusthasana

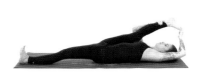

3 Supta Trivikramasana

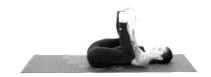

4 Ananda Balasana

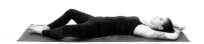

6 Supta Baddha Konasana

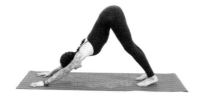

7 Adho Mukha Svanasana

8. *Uttanasana* (Standing Forward Fold)

9. *Utkatasana* (Chair Pose)

10. *Vrksasana* (Tree Pose)

11. *Virabhadrasana I* (Warrior I Pose)

12. *Virabhadrasana II* (Warrior II Pose)

13. *Trikonasana* (Triangle Pose)

14. *Ardha Chandrasana* (Balancing Half Moon Pose)

15. Repeat steps 7 through 14 on other side.

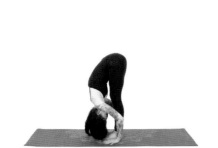

8 Uttanasana

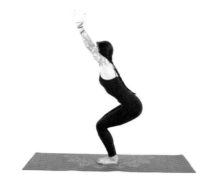

9 Utkatasana

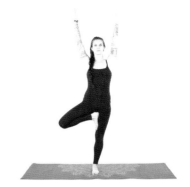

10 Vrksasana

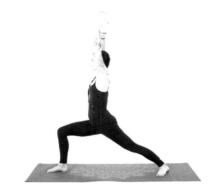

11 Virabhadrasana I

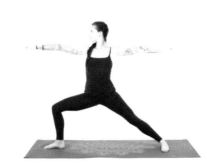

12 Virabhadrasana II

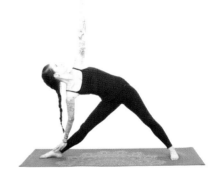

13 Trikonasana

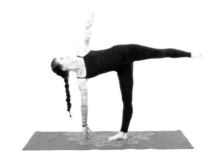

14 Ardha Chandrasana

Revolved Balancing Half Moon Pose
(Parivrtta Ardha Chandrasana)

This posture combines the warm-up postures of Balancing Half Moon (ARDHA CHANDRASANA) and Revolved Triangle Pose (PARIVRTTA TRIKONASANA). It integrates the openness and grounding of Revolved Triangle Pose with the lightness of Balancing Half Moon, creating balance and ease. Revolved Balancing Half Moon will feel less tough after practicing a sequence that strengthens the legs and core, opens the shoulders, and prepares for deep twists.

1. *SUPTA PADANGUSTHASANA* (Reclined Big Toe Pose)
2. *SUPTA TRIVIKRAMASANA* (Reclined Vishnu Pose)
3. *SUPTA PARIVRTTA PADANGUSTHASANA* (Reclining Revolved Hand-to-Big Toe Pose)
4. Repeat steps 1 through 3 on other side.
5. *SUPTA BADDHA KONASANA* (Reclined Bound Angle Pose)
6. Cat/Cow in Table Top
7. *SURYA NAMASKAR A* (Sun Salutation A—see page 1). Repeat 6 times.
8. *UTTANASANA* (Standing Forward Fold)
9. *UTKATASANA* (Chair Pose)

CONTINUED ON PAGE 20.

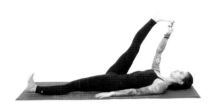

1   Supta Padangusthasana

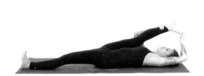

2   Supta Trivikramasana

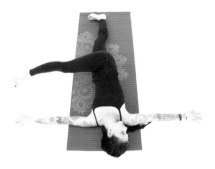

3   Supta Parivrtta
Padangusthasana

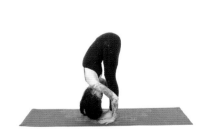

5   Supta Baddha Konasana

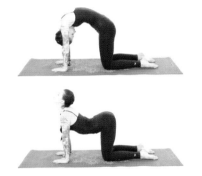

6   Cat/Cow in Table Top

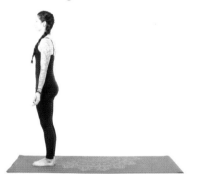

7   Sun Salutation A—see
page 1

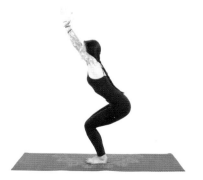

8   Uttanasana

9   Utkatasana

10. *Virabhadrasana I* (Warrior I Pose)

11. *Parsvottanasana* (Pyramid Pose)

12. *Alanasana* (High Lunge Pose)

13. *Parivrtta Alanasana* (Twisted High Lunge Pose)

14. *Virabhadrasana II* (Warrior II Pose)

15. *Trikonasana* (Triangle Pose)

16. *Ardha Chandrasana* (Balancing Half Moon Pose)

17. *Virabhadrasana III* (Warrior III Pose)

18. *Parivrtta Ardha Chandrasana* (Revolved Balancing Half Moon Pose)

19. Repeat steps 10 through 18 on other side.

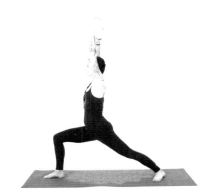

10 Virabhadrasana I

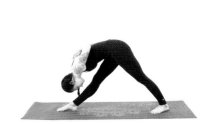

11 Parsvottanasana

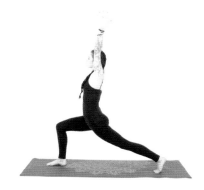

12 Alanasana

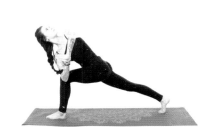

13 Parivrtta Alanasana

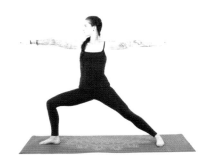

14 Virabhadrasana II

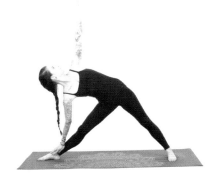

15 Trikonasana

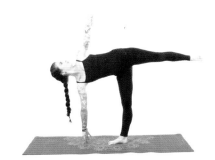

16 Ardha Chandrasana

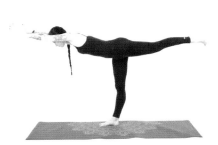

17 Virabhadrasana III

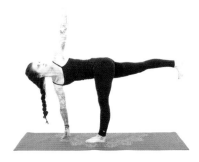

18 Parivrtta Ardha Chandrasana

Standing Hand-to-Big Toe Pose
(Utthita Hasta Padangusthasana)

The best way to get yourself prepared for this challenging standing balance is to practice it on your back. Use a strap during the supine warm-up sequence as well as the standing balance sequence until you can literally take your "hand to big toe." Speak no ill of your hamstrings and thank them regularly during this series. For runners, cyclists, and tall men (the world isn't built to your size, so I've heard), it can be quite an experience!

1. *Supta Padangusthasana* (Reclined Big Toe Pose)
2. *Supta Trivikramasana* (Reclined Vishnu Pose)
3. *Urdhva Mukha Paschimottanasana* (Upward Facing Forward Fold Pose)
4. Repeat steps 1 through 3 on other side.
5. *Paschimottanasana* (Seated Forward Fold)
6. *Baddha Konasana* (Bound Angle Pose)
7. *Anjaneyasana* (Knee Down Lunge)
8. *Ardha Hanumanasana* (Half Split Pose)
9. Repeat steps 7 and 8 on other side.
10. *Adho Mukha Svanasana* (Downward Facing Dog Pose)

Continued on page 24.

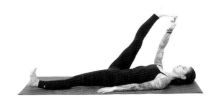

1   Supta Padangusthasana

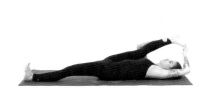

2   Supta Trivikramasana

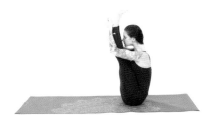

3   Urdhva Mukha Paschimottanasana

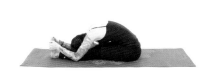

5   Paschimottanasana

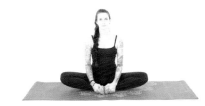

6   Baddha Konasana

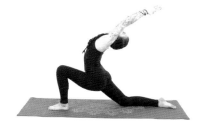

7   Anjaneyasana

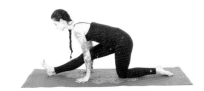

8   Ardha Hanumanasana

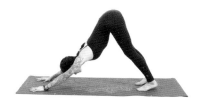

10   Adho Mukha Svanasana

11. *Surya Namaskar A* (Sun Salutation A—see page 1). Repeat 5 times.

12. *Uttanasana* (Standing Forward Fold)

13. *Vrksasana* (Tree Pose)

14. *Virabhadrasana I* (Warrior I Pose)

15. *Parsvottanasana* (Pyramid Pose)

16. *Alanasana* (High Lunge Pose)

17. *Virabhadrasana II* (Warrior II Pose)

18. *Trikonasana* (Triangle Pose)

19. Repeat steps 12 through 18 on other side.

20. *Utthita Hasta Padangusthasana* (Standing Hand-to-Big Toe Pose). Repeat on other side.

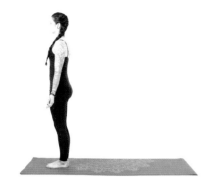

11 Sun Salutation
A—see page 1

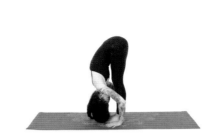

12 Uttanasana

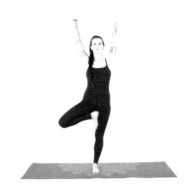

13 Vrksasana

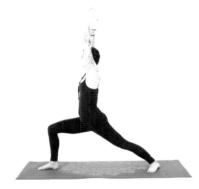

14 Virabhadrasana I

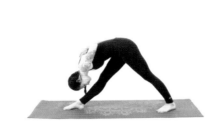

15 Parsvottanasana

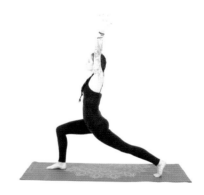

16 Alanasana

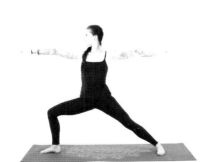

17 Virabhadrasana II

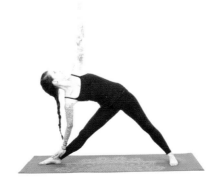

18 Trikonasana

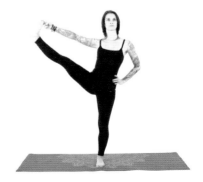

20 Utthita Hasta
Padangusthasana

Eagle Pose (Garudasana)

If you think of the double helix structure of our DNA strands, then you start to understand what is going on in Eagle Pose. The limbs wind around one another from ground to sky, massaging muscles and joints, and gaining balance and stability. If the upper back is very tight, modify by simply pressing the forearms into one another and thinking about broadening in between the shoulder blades.

1. *Janu Sirsasana* (Head to Knee Pose). Repeat on other side.
2. *Upavistha Konasana* (Seated Wide Angle Forward Bend)
3. *Adho Mukha Svanasana* (Downward Facing Dog Pose)
4. Forearm Plank. Hold for 1 minute to warm up shoulders.
5. *Purvottanasana* (Reverse Plank Pose)
6. *Baddha Virabhadrasana* (Humble Warrior Pose). Repeat on other side.
7. *Prasarita Padottanasana* (Standing Wide-Legged Forward Fold), with *Gomukhasana* (Cow Face Pose) bind in the arms, using a strap as you warm up. Repeat with opposite arm on top.
8. *Vrkasana* (Tree Pose). Repeat on other side.
9. *Garudasana* (Eagle Pose). Repeat on other side.

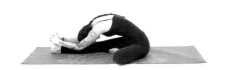

1 Janu Sirsasana

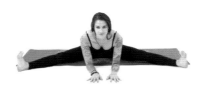

2 Upavistha Konasana

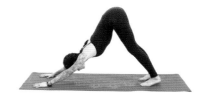

3 Adho Mukha Svanasana

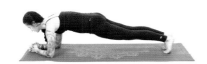

4 Forearm Plank

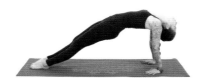

5 Purvottanasana

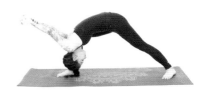

6 Baddha Virabhadrasana

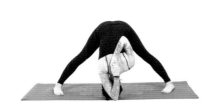

7 Prasarita Padottanasana
with Gomukhasana

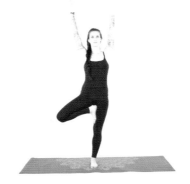

8 Vrksasana

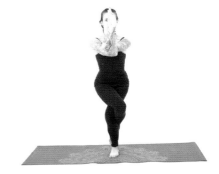

9 Garudasana

Bound Extended Side Angle Pose
(Baddha Utthita Parsvakonasana)

This is a variation that shows up often during the Power Yoga classes I teach and enjoy taking. Extended Side Angle, the old standby, plants one hand on the ground (either on a block or the floor) and extends the other toward the sky or parallel to the top ear. In the "bound" version, one arm snakes under the knee while the other moves around the back to perform a powerful heart and shoulder opener. While learning this pose, a strap can be used if the hands cannot clasp behind the hips or thigh.

1. *VIRASANA* (Hero Pose), with *GARUDASANA* (Eagle Pose) arms. Draw circles with elbows in both directions. Repeat with opposite arm on top.

2. *UPAVISTHA KONASANA* (Seated Wide Angle Forward Bend)

3. *JANU SIRSASANA* (Head to Knee Pose)

4. *PARIVRTTA JANU SIRSASANA* (Revolved Head to Knee Pose)

5. *BADDHA KONASANA* (Bound Angle Pose)

6. Repeat steps 3 and 4 on other side.

7. Cat/Cow in Table Top

8. *ADHO MUKHA SVANASANA* (Downward Facing Dog Pose)

CONTINUED ON PAGE 30.

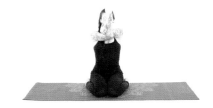

1 Virasana with
   Garudasana arms

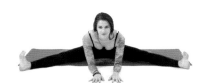

2 Upavistha Konasana

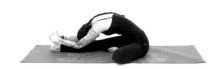

3 Janu Sirsasana

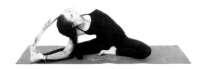

4 Parivrtta Janu Sirsasana

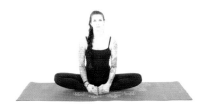

5 Baddha Konasana

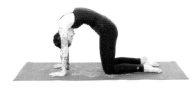

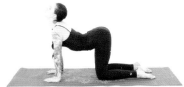

7 Cat/Cow in Table Top

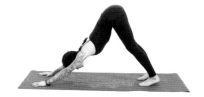

8 Adho Mukha Svanasana

9. *Virabhadrasana II* (Warrior II)

10. *Baddha Virabhadrasana* (Humble Warrior Pose)

11. *Viparita Virabhadrasana* (Peaceful Warrior Pose)

12. *Utthita Parsvakonasana* (Extended Side Angle Pose)

13. *Trikonasana* (Triangle Pose)

14. *Viparita Virabhadrasana* (Peaceful Warrior Pose)

15. Flow between steps 10 through 14 twice more, moving with the breath.

16. *Baddha Utthita Parsvakonasana* (Bound Extended Side Angle Pose)

17. Repeat steps 8 through 16 on other side.

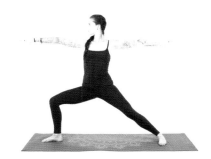

9 Virabhadrasana II

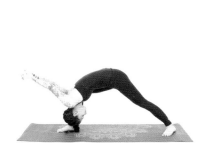

10 Baddha Virabhadrasana

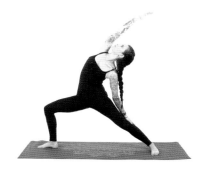

11 Viparita Virabhadrasana

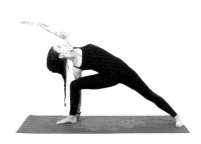

12 Utthita Parsvakonasana

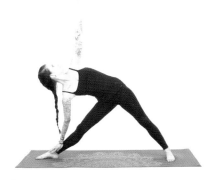

13 Trikonasana

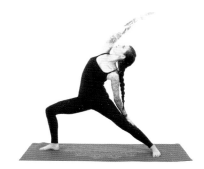

14 Viparita Virabhadrasana

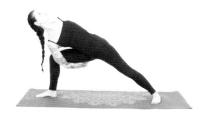

16 Baddha Utthita
Parsvakonasana

Bound Triangle Pose (Baddha Trikonasana)

Bound Triangle Pose is the middle child of a triumvirate of "Bound" poses: Bound Extended Side Angle, Bound Triangle, and, finally, Bird of Paradise Pose. For a long, powerful practice, start off with the sequence for *Baddha Utthita Parsvakonasana* (Bound Extended Side Angle) on page 28 and then continue on to this sequence (including the repeated poses) to build more heat in the legs and openness in the upper back, neck, and shoulders. Finally, move on to the next sequence, for Bird of Paradise Pose (*Svarga Dvijasana*) and enjoy the liftoff!

1. *Tadasana* (Mountain Pose)
2. *Garudasana* (Eagle Pose)
3. *Virabhadrasana III* (Warrior III Pose)
4. *Virabhadrasana I* (Warrior I Pose)
5. *Baddha Virabhadrasana* (Humble Warrior Pose)
6. *Virabhadrasana II* (Warrior II Pose)
7. *Viparita Virabhadrasana* (Peaceful Warrior Pose)

Continued on page 34.

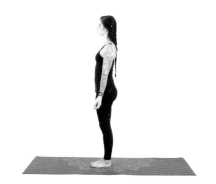

1 Tadasana

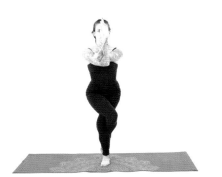

2 Garudasana

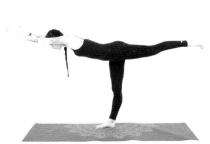

3 Virabhadrasana III

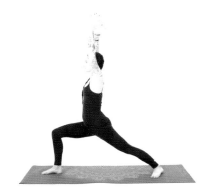

4 Virabhadrasana I

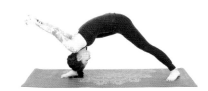

5 Baddha Virabhadrasana

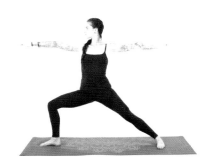

6 Virabhadrasana II

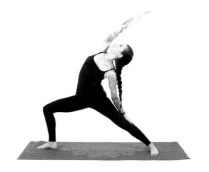

7 Viparita Virabhadrasana

8. *Trikonasana* (Triangle Pose)

9. *Virabhadrasana II* (Warrior II Pose)

10. *Adho Mukha Svanasana* (Downward Facing Dog Pose)

11. Repeat steps 1 through 10 on other side. Repeat both sides as a flow 2 more times to build heat.

12. *Prasarita Padottanasana* (Standing Wide-Legged Forward Fold). Note: Repeat a second time with hands interlaced behind the lower back.

13. *Virabhadrasana* II (Warrior II Pose)

14. *Baddha Utthita Parsvakonasana* (Bound Extended Side Angle Pose)

15. *Baddha Trikonasana* (Bound Triangle Pose)

16. Repeat steps 13 through 15 on other side.

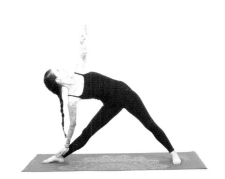

8 Trikonasana

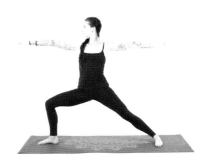

9 Virabhadrasana II

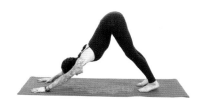

10 Adho Mukha Svanasana

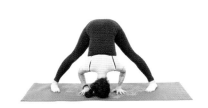

12 Prasarita Padottanasana

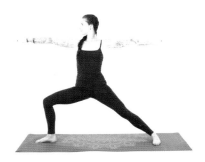

13 Virabhadrasana II

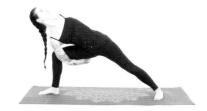

14 Baddha Utthita
Parsvakonasana

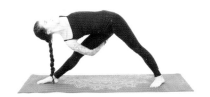

15 Baddha Trikonasana

Bird of Paradise Pose (Svarga Dvijasana)

Take flight into this beautiful and challenging standing balance! This pose serves as a transition from the grounding poses in this chapter to the gravity-defying poses in the chapter that follows. The firmness of the standing leg allows the heart to shine forward and the extended leg to touch the sky. As with many of these postures, the key to this pose is patience. If the knees, shoulders, or hips start to feel discomfort or pain, meet yourself where you are and enjoy more time in the practice of Grounding Down before the practice of flight.

1. *Supta Baddha Konasana* (Reclined Bound Angle Pose)

2. *Janu Sirsasana* (Head to Knee Pose)

3. *Parivrtta Janu Sirsasana* (Revolved Seated Head to Knee Pose)

4. Repeat steps 2 and 3 on other side.

5. *Paschimottanasana* (Seated Forward Fold)

6. *Upavistha Konasana* (Seated Wide Angle Forward Bend)

7. *Surya Namaskar A* (Sun Salutation A—see page 1). Repeat 5 times.

8. *Yoga Mudrasana, variation* (Standing Forward Fold with Hands Interlaced Behind Back). Hold for 2–3 minutes.

Continued on page 38.

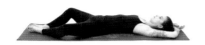

1 Supta Baddha Konasana

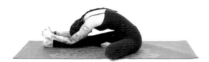

2 Janu Sirsasana

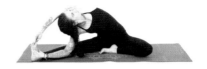

3 Parivrtta Janu Sirsasana

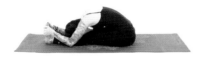

5 Paschimottanasana

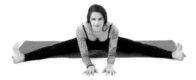

6 Upavistha Konasana

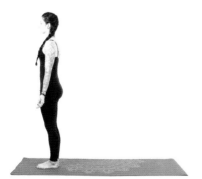

7 Sun Salutation A—
   see page 1

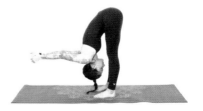

8 Yoga Mudrasana

9.   *Malasana* (Seated Squat Pose)

10. *Vrksasana* (Tree Pose). Repeat on other side.

11. *Utthita Hasta Padangusthasana* (Standing Hand-to-Big Toe Pose). Repeat on other side.

12. *Virabhadrasana II* (Warrior II Pose)

13.   *Baddha Utthita Parsvakonasana* (Bound Extended Side Angle Pose)

14. *Trikonasana* (Triangle Pose). Note: If you can, move into *Baddha Trikonasana*.

15.   *Svarga Dvijasana* (Bird of Paradise Pose)

16. Repeat steps 12 through 15 on other side.

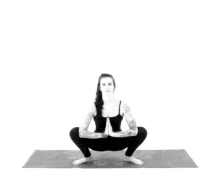

9 Malasana

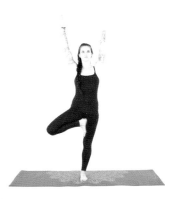

10 Vrksasana

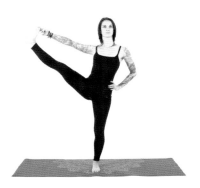

11 Utthita Hasta Padangusthasana

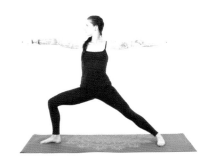

12 Virabhadrasana II

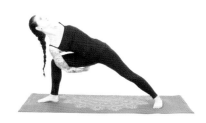

13 Baddha Utthita Parsvakonasana

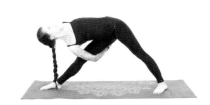

14 Baddha Trikonasana

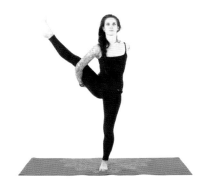

15 Svarga Dvijasana

Take Flight

Arm Balancing Poses

"Jump Backs"

"Jump Back" is the term used in some styles of yoga to describe the motion of jumping from *Ardha Uttanasana* or *Uttanasana* (Half or Full Standing Forward Fold Pose) directly into *Chaturanga Dandasana* (Four-Limbed Staff Pose). In Ashtanga Yoga classes, a "jump back" is used anytime the yogi transitions from a seated posture directly into a *Chaturanga Dandasana*, seeming to float through the air as they do. Developing the strength and coordination to execute this movement takes time and patience, but here's a sequence to help get you on your way!

1. *Sukhasana* (Easy Pose). Note: Practice 2–3 sets of *Kapalabhati Pranayama* (Skull Shining Breath) if it's a part of your yoga practice.

2. *Uddiyana Bandha* (Upward Abdominal Lock). Hold for 5–10 seconds; repeat 5 times.

3. *Surya Namaskar A* (Sun Salutation A—see page 1). Repeat 5 times.

4. *Surya Namaskar B* (Sun Salutation B—see page 2). Repeat 5 times.

5. *Navasana* (Boat Pose)

6. *Balasana* (Child's Pose)

7. *Tolasana* (Scale Pose). Rest afterward for 5 cycles of breath.

8. *Bakasana* (Crow Pose). Rest afterward for 5 cycles of breath.

9. *Ardha Matsyendrasana* (Half Seated Twist Pose). Repeat on the other side.

10. "Jump Backs": Practice another 5 *Surya Namaskar A* (Sun Salutation A—see page 1), using core strength and pelvic floor lift to jump from *Uttanasana* (Standing Forward Fold) directly into *Chaturanga Dandasana* (Four-Limbed Staff Pose).

11. *Lolasana* (Pendant Pose).

12. Jump back from this posture directly into *Chaturanga Dandasana*. Repeat 3 times.

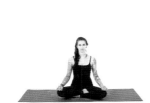

1   Sukhasana

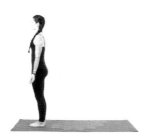

3   Sun Salutation A—
see page 1

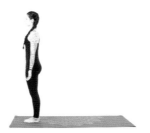

4   Sun Salutation B—
see page 2

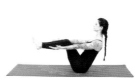

5   Navasana

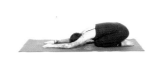

6   Balasana

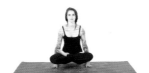

7   Tolasana

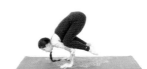

8   Bakasana

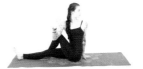

9   Ardha
Matsyendrasana

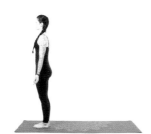

10   Sun Salutation A—
see page 1

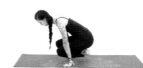

11   Lolasana

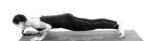

12   Chaturanga
Dandasana

Four-Limbed Staff Pose (Chaturanga Dandasana)

Even students with years of yoga practice under their belt (or, rather, spandex pants) still find challenge in this posture. In and of itself, CHATURANGA DANDASANA is not an arm balance—but it is integral to developing a stronger arm balance practice. Although CHATURANGA DANDASANA does not require significant warm up, here are some poses that can help develop the strength needed to feel steady.

1. ADHO MUKHA SVANASANA (Downward Facing Dog Pose)
2. Plank Pose. Flow between steps 1 and 2 five times, moving with the breath.
3. Plank Pose. Hold for 1–2 minutes.
4. BALASANA (Child's Pose)
5. BHUJANGASANA (Cobra Pose)
6. URDHVA MUKHA SVANASANA (Upward Facing Dog Pose). Flow between steps 4 and 6, moving with the breath.
7. BALASANA (Child's Pose)
8. Forearm Plank Pose. Hold for 1–2 minutes.
9. DANDASANA (Staff Pose)
10. Practice CHATURANGA DANDASANA (Four Limbed Staff Pose) against a wall, standing a few inches from the wall and finding the alignment you would otherwise find on the floor. Note: This is also a great modification to use for prenatal yoga!

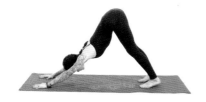

1   Adho Mukha Svanasana

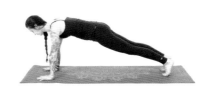

2   Plank

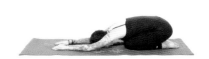

4   Balasana

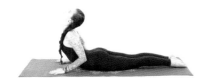

5   Bhujangasana

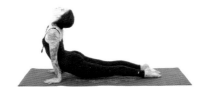

6   Urdhva Mukha Svanasana

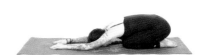

7   Balasana

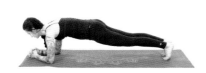

8   Forearm Plank

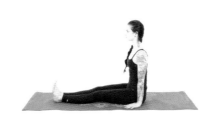

9   Dandasana

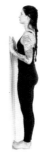

10   Chaturanga Dandasana

Side Plank Pose (Vasisthasana)

As with many of the poses we work toward, there is a modification available that is excellent for most levels of yoga students. This sequence will offer two stages: you can stop at the first *Vasisthasana* and enjoy all of the benefits this pose provides. The first version of the pose is essentially Mountain Pose, or *Tadasana*, on its side. Like in Mountain Pose, we stack our body parts to minimize effort and strengthen the bones. Alternately, you can continue from there to the full version of the pose, where the top leg is extended to the sky until it is perpendicular to the floor.

1. *Supta Padangusthasana* (Reclined Big Toe Pose)
2. *Supta Trivikramasana* (Reclined Vishnu Pose)
3. *Urdhva Mukha Paschimottanasana* (Upward Facing Forward Fold Pose)
4. Repeat steps 1–3 on other side.
5. *Upavistha Konasana* (Seated Wide Angle Forward Bend)
6. *Baddha Konasana* (Bound Angle Pose)
7. *Adho Mukha Svanasana* (Downward Facing Dog Pose)
8. *Surya Namaskar A* (Sun Salutation A—see page 1). Repeat 5 times.
9. *Bhujangasana* (Cobra Pose)
10. Sphinx Pose
11. *Balasana* (Child's Pose)
12. Plank Pose

Continued on page 48.

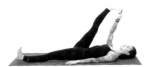

1 Supta
Padangusthasana

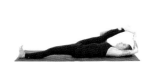

2 Supta
Trivikramasana

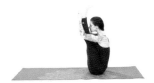

3 Urdhva Mukha
Paschimottanasana

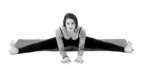

5 Upavistha
Konasana

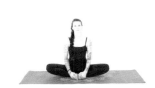

6 Baddha Konasana

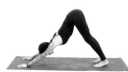

7 Adho Mukha
Svanasana

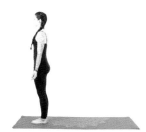

8 Sun Salutation A—
see page 1

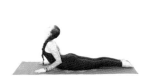

9 Bhujangasana

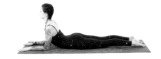

10 Sphinx

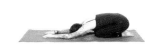

11 Balasana

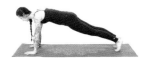

12 Plank

13. *Vasisthasana I* (Side Plank Pose). Hold for 5 cycles of breath and repeat on other side.

14. *Uttanasana* (Standing Forward Fold). Note: Take hands to opposite elbow to release the upper back muscles.

15. *Vrksasana* (Tree Pose). Repeat on other side.

16. *Utthita Hasta Padangusthasana* (Standing Hand-to-Big Toe Pose). Repeat on other side.

17. *Virabhadrasana I* (Warrior I Pose)

18. *Virabhadrasana II* (Warrior II Pose)

19. *Trikonasana* (Triangle Pose)

20. *Ardha Chandrasana* (Balancing Half Moon Pose)

21. *Virabhadrasana II* (Warrior II Pose)

22. Plank Pose

23. *Vasisthasana II* (Side Plank Pose), with option to extend top leg to sky.

24. Repeat steps 17 through 23 on other side.

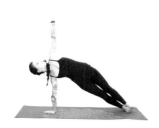

13 Vasisthasana I

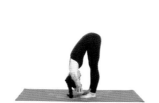

14 Uttanasana

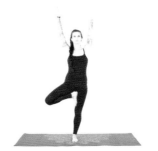

15 Vrksasana

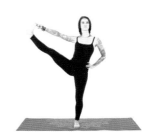

16 Utthita Hasta Padangusthasana

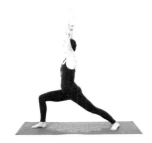

17 Virabhadrasana I

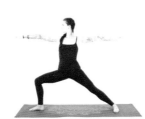

18 Virabhadrasana II

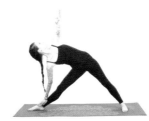

19 Trikonasana

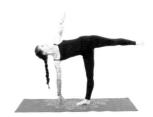

20 Ardha Chandrasana

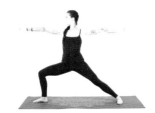

21 Virabhadrasana II

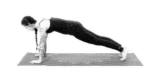

22 Plank

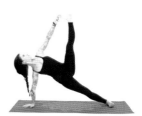

23 Vasisthasana II

Tiger Pose (Vyaghrasana)

This is a great introduction to arm balancing. It helps set the foundation for more complex arm balances by teaching us how to firm the core, engage the hand and arm muscles, and reduce pressure on the wrists. That said, it's pretty low risk. Falling looks a lot like gently tipping to the floor. Yoga teacher secret: this pose is even more fun with a little Tiger ROAR.

1. Cat/Cow in Table Top. Note: Get used to feeling the forearm muscles engage upward while pressing into the finger pads.
2. *Parighasana* (Gate Pose). Repeat on other side.
3. *Bhujangasana* (Cobra Pose). Repeat 3 times, with rests in between.
4. *Dhanurasana* (Bow Pose). Note: Have this be a gentle bow, not your fullest expression.
5. *Balasana* (Child's Pose)
6. *Ardha Matsyendrasana* (Half Seated Twist Pose). Repeat on other side.
7. *Vyaghrasana* (Tiger Pose). Repeat on other side.

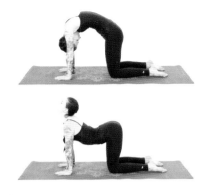

1   Cat/Cow in Table Top

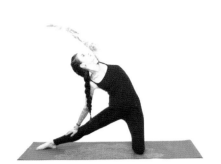

2   Parighasana

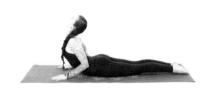

3   Bhujangasana

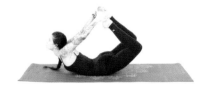

4   Dhanurasana

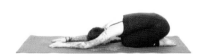

5   Balasana

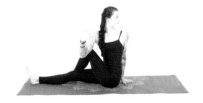

6   Ardha Matsyendrasana

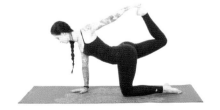

7   Vyaghrasana

Scale Pose (*Tolasana*)

If you cannot practice *Padmasana* (Lotus Pose) without knee pain (or discomfort in general), then try to move into *Tolasana* (Scale Pose) from *Sukhasana* (Easy Pose). You can even keep the outer edge of the lower foot down on the ground as you lift the rest of your body; blocks underneath the hands provide great support, too. Warning: practicing this pose regularly may result in Superhero Abs, super-strong shoulders, and smoother "Jump Backs."

1. *Sukhasana* (Easy Pose). Note: Practice 2–3 sets of *Kapalabhati Pranayama* (Skull Shining Breath) if it's a part of your yoga practice.

2. *Uddiyana Bandha* (Upward Abdominal Lock). Hold for 5–10 seconds, repeat 5 times.

3. *Ardha Matsyendrasana* (Half Seated Twist Pose). Repeat on other side.

4. *Baddha Konasana* (Bound Angle Pose)

5. *Upavistha Konasana* (Seated Wide Angle Forward Bend)

6. *Surya Namaskar A* (Sun Salutation A—see page 1). Repeat 5 times.

7. *Yoga Mudrasana, variation* (Standing Forward Fold with Hands Interlaced Behind Back)

8. *Virasana* (Hero Pose), with *Garudasana* (Eagle Pose) arms. Draw circles with elbows in both directions. Repeat with opposite arm on top.

9. *Janu Sirsasana* (Head to Knee Pose)

10. *Parivrtta Janu Sirsasana* (Revolved Head to Knee Pose)

11. Repeat steps 9 and 10 on other side.

12. *Tolasana* (Scale Pose)

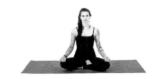

1 Sukhasana

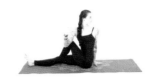

3 Ardha Matsyendrasana

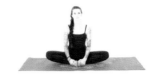

4 Baddha Konasana

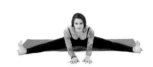

5 Upavistha Konasana

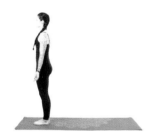

6 Sun Salutation A—see page 1

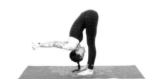

7 Yoga Mudrasana

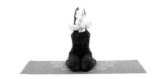

8 Virasana with Garudasana arms

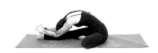

9 Janu Sirsasana

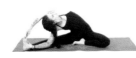

10 Parivrtta Janu Sirsasana

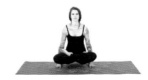

12 Tolasana

Crow Pose (Bakasana)

Ever heard the phrase *A WATCHED POT NEVER BOILS*? In *BAKASANA* (Crow Pose), watched feet never lift. Let both your gaze and your core lift up and your feet will follow.

1. *UTTANASANA* (Standing Forward Fold Pose)
2. Take your hands to a block or to the floor about six inches in front of your feet. Shift your weight forward to your hands by lifting your heels and tailbone, then shift the weight back to your feet and lower the heels. Repeat 6–12 times. Feel the belly lift and the core engage as you shift forward.
3. *SURYA NAMASKAR A* (Sun Salutation A—see page 1). Repeat 5 times.
4. *UTKATASANA* (Chair Pose) Note: Practice the first Chair Pose with a block in between the thighs, engaging in toward the block. Hold for 5 cycles of breath.
5. Lower to *NAVASANA* (Boat Pose).
6. Repeat steps 4 and 5 two additional times.
7. Cat/Cow in Table Top
8. Plank Pose
9. *VASISTHASANA I* (Side Plank Pose). Repeat on other side.
10. *BALASANA* (Child's Pose)
11. *PRASARITA PADOTTANASANA* (Standing Wide-Legged Forward Fold)
12. *MALASANA* (Garland Pose)
13. *BAKASANA* (Crow Pose)

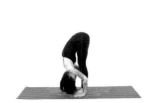

1 Uttanasana

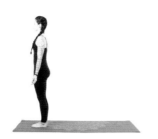

3 Sun Salutation A—
see page 1

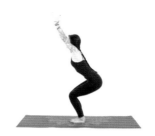

4 Utkatasana

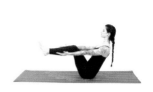

5 Navasana

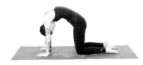

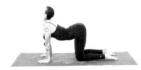

7 Cat/Cow in
Table Top

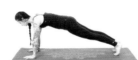

8 Plank

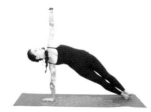

9 Vasisthasana I

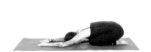

10 Balasana

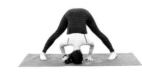

11 Prasarita
Padottanasana

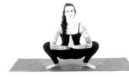

12 Malasana

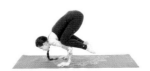

13 Bakasana

Side Crow Pose (Parsva Bakasana)

Am I the only one who finds Side Crow Pose more accessible than Crow Pose (*Bakasana*)? Maybe it's just that the ground seems closer, so I'm less worried about face-planting from trepidation-inducing heights. In either pose, placing a block or a pillow in front of the face helps get past that road block. Now you just have to get your feet off the floor . . .

1. *Jathara Parivartanasana* (Revolved Abdomen Pose). Flow from side to side with the breath, building fire in the core.
2. *Ardha Matsyendrasana* (Half Seated Twist Pose). Repeat on other side.
3. *Utkatasana* (Chair Pose)
4. *Parivrtta Utkatasana* (Revolved Chair Pose). Repeat other side.
5. *Utkatasana* (Chair Pose)
6. Lower to *Prapadasana* (Tiptoe Pose). Keep the knees and thighs hugging together, rise back to *Utkasasana*.
7. Repeat steps 5 and 6 three times.
8. *Surya Namaskar A* (Sun Salutation A—see page 1). Repeat 5 times.
9. *Balasana* (Child's Pose)
10. Plank Pose
11. *Chaturanga Dandasana* (Four-Limbed Staff Pose)
12. Repeat steps 10 and 11 three times.
13. *Balasana* (Child's Pose)
14. *Parsva Bakasana* (Side Crow Pose). Repeat other side.

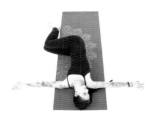

1 Jathara
Parivartanasana

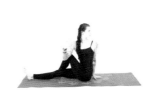

2 Ardha
Matsyendrasana

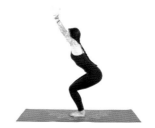

3 Utkatasana

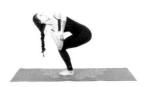

4 Parivrtta
Utkatasana

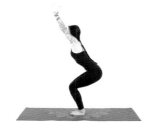

5 Utkatasana

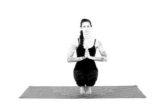

6 Prapadasana

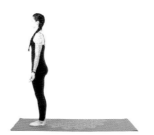

8 Sun Salutation A—
see page 1

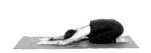

9 Balasana

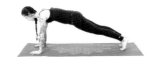

10 Plank

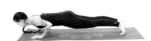

11 Chaturanga
Dandasana

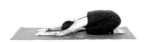

13 Balasana

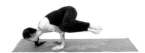

14 Parsva Bakasana

Firefly Pose (*Tittibhasana*)

Do you know why I love Firefly Pose? Because instead of worrying about falling on my face, I know that, if worse comes to worst, all that can happen is I'll fall on my butt. Seeing as that happens pretty often anyway, I'm pretty secure in doing it even more often as I try to master this pose.

1. *Setu Bandhasana* (Bridge Pose)
2. *Ananda Balasana* (Happy Baby Pose)
3. *Virasana* (Hero Pose), with *Garudasana* (Eagle Pose) arms. Draw circles with elbows in both directions. Repeat with opposite arm on top.
4. *Paschimottanasana* (Seated Forward Fold)
5. *Upavistha Konasana* (Seated Wide Angle Forward Bend)
6. *Ardha Matsyendrasana* (Half Seated Twist Pose). Repeat on other side.
7. *Baddha Konasana* (Bound Angle Pose)
8. *Surya Namaskar A* (Sun Salutation A—see page 1). Repeat 5 times.
9. *Balasana* (Child's Pose)

Continued on page 60.

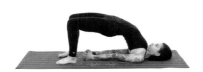

1 Setu Bandhasana

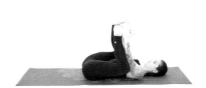

2 Ananda Balasana

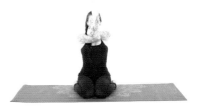

3 Virasana with Garudasana arms

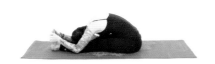

4 Paschimottanasana

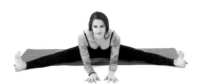

5 Upavistha Konasana

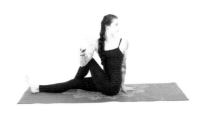

6 Ardha Matsyendrasana

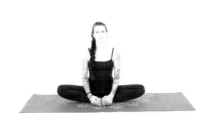

7 Baddha Konasana

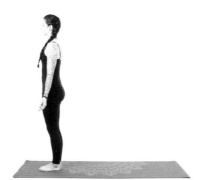

8 Sun Salutation A—see page 1

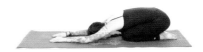

9 Balasana

10. *Janu Sirsasana* (Head to Knee Pose)

11. *Parivrtta Janu Sirsasana* (Revolved Head to Knee Pose)

12. Repeat steps 10 and 11 on other side.

13. *Prasarita Padottanasana* (Standing Wide-Legged Forward Fold)

14. *Deviasana* (Goddess Pose)

15. *Malasana* (Garland Pose)

16. *Navasana* (Boat Pose)

17. *Bakasana* (Crow Pose)

18. *Tittibhasana* (Firefly Pose)

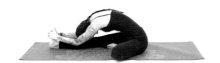

10 Janu Sirsasana

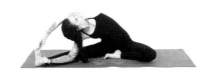

11 Parivrtta Janu Sirsasana

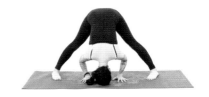

13 Prasarita Padottanasana

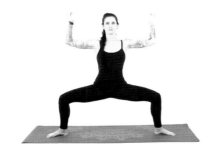

14 Deviasana

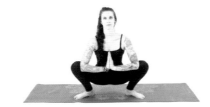

15 Malasana

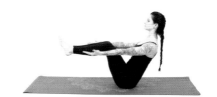

16 Navasana

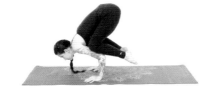

17 Bakasana

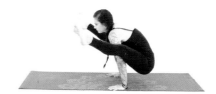

18 Tittibhasana

Flying Pigeon Pose (Eka Pada Galavasana)

One week, as I taught this pose, two men with significant upper body strength (neither of whom had ever tried Flying Pigeon before), muscled their way into it on the first try, no problem. I, on the other hand, had attempted this posture for years, falling over like a true Yoga Champion before my legs left the ground for a hot second. With patience, however, comes a truly beautiful posture well worth the effort.

1. *Surya Namaskar A* (Sun Salutation A—see page 1). Repeat 5 times.
2. *Surya Namaskar B* (Sun Salutation B—see page 2). Repeat 5 times.
3. *Balasana* (Child's Pose)
4. Plank Pose
5. *Chaturanga Dandasana* (Four-Limbed Staff Pose)
6. Repeat steps 4 and 5 three times.
7. *Balasana* (Child's Pose)
8. *Prasarita Padottanasana* (Standing Wide-Legged Forward Fold)
9. *Malasana* (Garland Pose)

Continued on page 64.

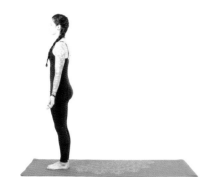

1 Sun Salutation A— see page 1

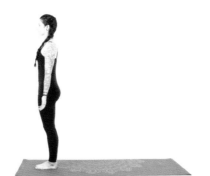

2 Sun Salutation B—see page 2

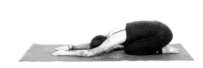

3 Balasana

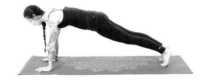

4 Plank

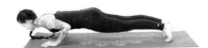

5 Chaturanga Dandasana

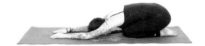

7 Balasana

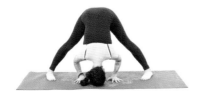

8 Prasarita Padottanasana

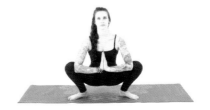

9 Malasana

63

10. *Bakasana* (Crow Pose)

11. *Supta Eka Pada Rajakapotasana* (Resting Pigeon Pose). Repeat other side.

12. *Adho Mukha Svanasana* (Downward Facing Dog Pose). Extend one leg back into the air for "Three-Legged Dog." Hold for 5 cycles of breath and repeat on the other side.

13. *Vrksasana* (Tree Pose). Repeat on other side.

14. *Virabhadrasana III* (Warrior III Pose). Repeat on other side.

15. *Tadasana* (Mountain Pose)

16. *Utkatasana* (Chair Pose). Cross your right ankle over your left knee.

17. *Eka Pada Galavasana* (Flying Pigeon Pose)

18. Repeat steps 15 through 17 on other side.

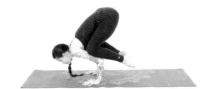

10 Bakasana

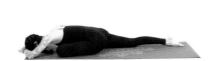

11 Supta Eka Pada
Rajakapotasana

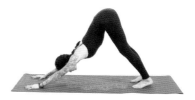

12 Adho Mukha Svanasana

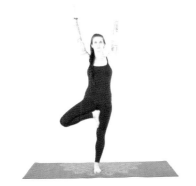

13 Vrksasana

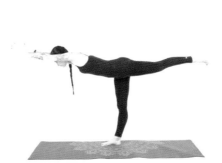

14 Virabhadrasana III

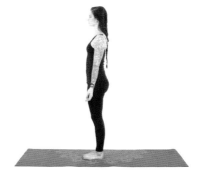

15 Tadasana

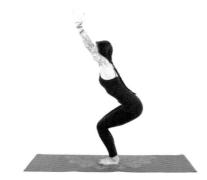

16 Utkatasana

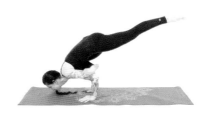

17 Eka Pada Galavasana

Pose Dedicated to the Sage Koundinya II
(Eka Pada Koundinyasana II)

Like Flying Pigeon Pose, I worked on this pose for years before anything remotely interesting happened. *Koundinyasana I* is entered from *Parsva Bakasana* (Side Crow) by extending both legs like scissors. To try *Koundinyasana I*, use the same warm-up sequence as *Parsva Bakasana*. For *Koundinyasana II*, it's a whole new ball game, with a new set of poses to match!

1. *Supta Padangusthasana* (Reclined Big Toe Pose)
2. *Supta Trivikramasana* (Reclined Vishnu Pose)
3. *Urdhva Mukha Paschimottanasana* (Upward Facing Forward Fold Pose)
4. Repeat steps 1 and 2 on other side.
5. *Ananda Balasana* (Happy Baby Pose)
6. Cat/Cow in Table Top
7. *Anjaneyasana* (Knee Down Lunge)
8. *Ardha Hanumanasana* (Half Split Pose)
9. Flow between steps 7 and 8.
10. *Surya Namaskar B* (Sun Salutation B—see page 2). Repeat 5 times.
11. Plank Pose
12. *Chaturanga Dandasana* (Four-Limbed Staff Pose)

Continued on page 68.

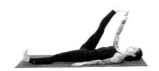

1 Supta
Padangusthasana

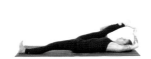

2 Supta
Trivikramasana

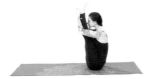

3 Urdhva Mukha
Paschimottanasana

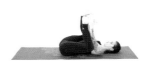

5 Ananda Balasana

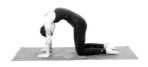
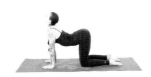

6 Cat/Cow in
Table Top

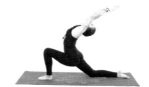

7 Anjaneyasana

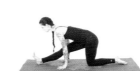

8 Ardha
Hanumanasana

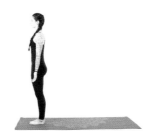

10 Sun Salutation B—
see page 2

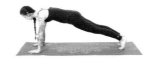

11 Plank

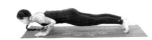

12 Chaturanga
Dandasana

13. Repeat steps 11 and 12 three times.

14. *Balasana* (Child's Pose)

15. *Paschimottanasana* (Seated Forward Fold)

16. *Virabhadrasana II* (Warrior II Pose)

17. *Trikonasana* (Triangle Pose)

18. *Prasarita Padottanasana* (Standing Wide-Legged Forward Fold)

19. Repeat steps 16 and 17 on other side.

20. *Malasana* (Garland Pose)

21. *Bakasana* (Crow Pose)

22. *Adho Mukha Svanasana* (Downward Facing Dog Pose)

23. *Eka Pada Koundinyasana II* (Pose Dedicated to the Sage Koundinya II). Repeat on other side.

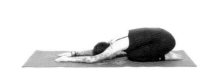

14 Balasana

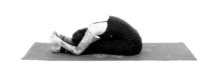

15 Paschimottanasana

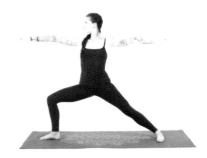

16 Virabhadrasana II

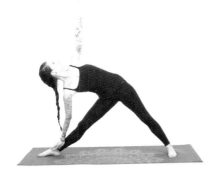

17 Trikonasana

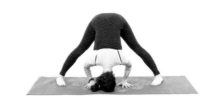

18 Prasarita Padottanasana

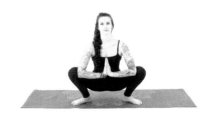

20 Malasana

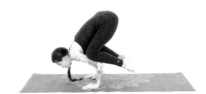

21 Bakasana

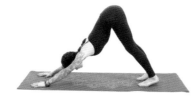

22 Adho Mukha Svanasana

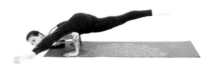

23 Eka Pada
Koundinyasana II

Open Up

Back Bends and Heart Openers

"Wild Thing" (Camatkarasana)

This pose, sometimes called "Flip Dog" (or some variation of that title), is entered into from a leg extension in Downward Facing Dog and lands in the "seems scarier than it is" category. As we practice yoga more often, we develop a clearer sense of where our bodies are in space (a.k.a. proprioception), and poses like "Wild Thing" start to feel safer. Trust that the floor will be there to catch you and open your heart to the sky.

1. Cat/Cow in Table Top
2. *Vyaghrasana* (Tiger Pose). Repeat other side.
3. *Surya Namaskar A* (Sun Salutation A—see page 1). Repeat 5 times.
4. *Bhujangasana* (Cobra Pose)
5. *Salabhasana* (Locust Pose)
6. *Dhanurasana* (Bow Pose)
7. *Balasana* (Child's Pose)
8. *Adho Mukha Svanasana* (Downward Facing Dog Pose)
9. *Camatkarasana* ("Wild Thing"). Repeat on other side.

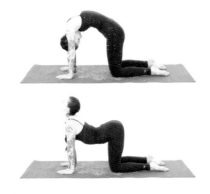

1 Cat/Cow in Table Top

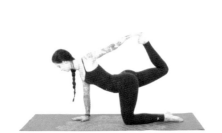

2 Vyaghrasana

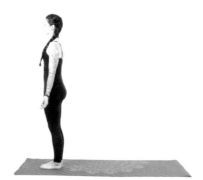

3 Sun Salutation A—
see page 1

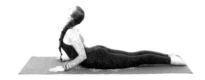

4 Bhujangasana

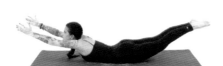

5 Salabhasana

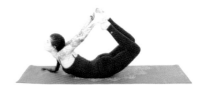

6 Dhanurasana

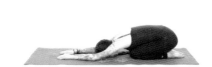

7 Balasana

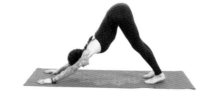

8 Adho Mukha Svanasana

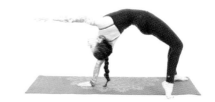

9 Camatkarasana

Reverse Plank Pose (Purvottanasana)

I like teaching Reverse Plank Pose during classes that incorporate a lot of *Vinyasas*. It helps strengthen and stretch out the wrists while simultaneously lengthening the entire front of the body. For a little something extra, stick out your tongue during Reverse Plank for *Simhasana Pranayama* (Lion's Breath)—do your best Gene Simmons impression!

1. *Supta Virasana* (Reclined Hero Pose). Note: Come into the restorative version of this pose, using as many pillows as you like behind the back. If this pose doesn't work for your knees, come into *Supta Baddha Konasana* (Reclined Bound Angle Pose).

2. *Balasana* (Child's Pose)

3. Cat/Cow in Table Top

4. *Uttanasana* (Standing Forward Fold)

5. *Urdhva Hastasana* (Upward Hands Pose)

6. *Yoga Mudrasana, variation* (Standing Forward Fold with Hands Interlaced Behind Back)

7. *Adho Mukha Svanasana* (Downward Facing Dog Pose)

Continued on page 76.

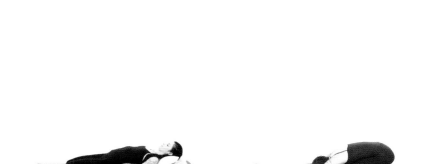

1   Supta Virasana

2   Balasana

3   Cat/Cow in Table Top

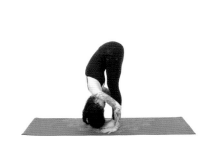

4   Uttanasana

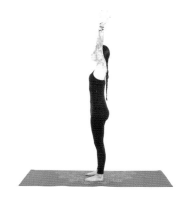

5   Urdhva Hastasana

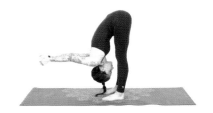

6   Yoga Mudrasana

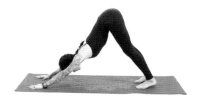

7   Adho Mukha Svanasana

8. *Urdhva Mukha Svanasana* (Upward Facing Dog Pose)

9. Repeat steps 7 and 8 five times, flowing between the two postures.

10. *Paschimottanasana* (Seated Forward Fold)

11. Reverse Table Top

12. *Baddha Konasana* (Bound Angle Pose)

13. *Setu Bandhasana* (Bridge Pose)

14. *Dandasana* (Staff Pose)

15. *Purvottanasana* (Reverse Plank Pose)

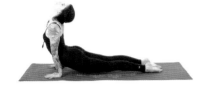

8 Urdhva Mukha Svanasana

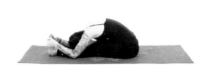

10 Paschimottanasana

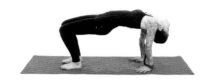

11 Reverse Table Top

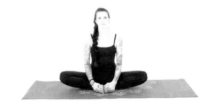

12 Baddha Konasana

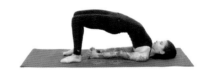

13 Setu Bandhasana

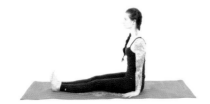

14 Dandasana

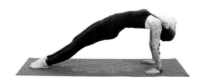

15 Purvottanasana

Fish Pose (Matsyasana)

Traditionally, this pose is entered into with the legs crossed in PADMASANA (Lotus Pose). I don't think that having that leg position is particularly relevant to the heart-opening therapeutic aspects of Fish Pose, though. In this sequence, keep the legs extended.

1. *SUPTA BADDHA KONASANA* (Reclined Bound Angle Pose)
2. *SETU BANDHASANA* (Bridge Pose)
3. *ANANDA BALASANA* (Happy Baby Pose)
4. Cat/Cow in Table Top
5. *BHUJANGASANA* (Cobra Pose)
6. *SALABHASANA* (Locust Pose)
7. *DHANURASANA* (Bow Pose)
8. *BALASANA* (Child's Pose)

CONTINUED ON PAGE 80.

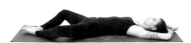

1 Supta Baddha Konasana

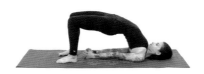

2 Setu Bandhasana

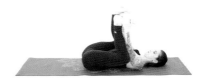

3 Ananda Balasana

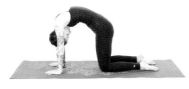
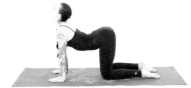

4 Cat/Cow in Table Top

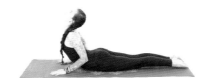

5 Bhujangasana

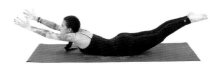

6 Salabhasana

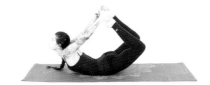

7 Dhanurasana

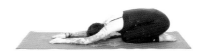

8 Balasana

9. *Adho Mukha Svanasana* (Downward Facing Dog Pose)
10. *Yoga Mudrasana, variation* (Standing Forward Fold with Hands Interlaced Behind Back)
11. Reverse Table Top
12. *Baddha Konasana* (Bound Angle Pose)
13. *Salamba Sarvangasana* (Shoulderstand Pose)
14. *Halasana* (Plow Pose)
15. *Matsyasana* (Fish Pose)

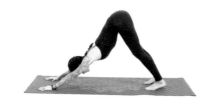

9 Adho Mukha Svanasana

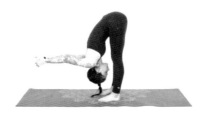

10 Yoga Mudrasana

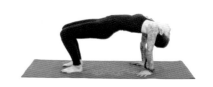

11 Reverse Table Top

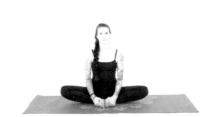

12 Baddha Konasana

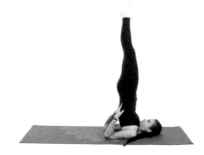

13 Salamba Sarvangasana

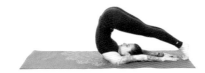

14 Halasana

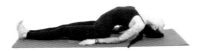

15 Matsyasana

Camel Pose (Ustrasana)

Sometimes, I devote an entire class to the magnificence that is Camel Pose. There are just so many interesting ways to explore the posture. I like practicing it with my thighs and hipbones pressing into a wall and my hands on my lower back. Other times, I'll teach the pose with hands together in front of the heart in a prayer position. As your spine gains flexibility, place blocks to the outside of your feet and lower your hands to the blocks during the back bend; eventually, the hands may comfortably reach the feet.

1. *BALASANA* (Child's Pose)

2. Cat/Cow in Table Top

3. *ANJANEYASANA* (Knee Down Lunge)

4. *ARDHA HANUMANASANA* (Half Split Pose)

5. *VYAGHRASANA* (Tiger Pose)

6. Repeat steps 2 through 5 on other side

7. *SURYA NAMASKAR B* (Sun Salutation B—see page 2). Repeat 5 times, substituting *ALANASANA* (High Lunge Pose) for *VIRABHADRASANA I* (Warrior I).

8. *TADASANA* (Mountain Pose). Note: Take your hands to your lower back for a standing version of *USTRASANA* (Camel Pose).

9. *YOGA MUDRASANA, VARIATION* (Standing Forward Fold with Hands Interlaced Behind Back)

CONTINUED ON PAGE 84.

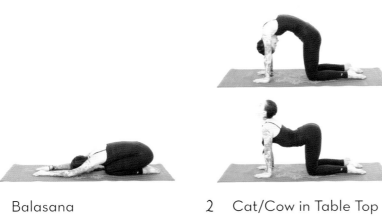

1   Balasana

2   Cat/Cow in Table Top

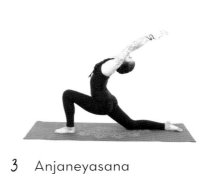

3   Anjaneyasana

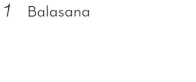

4   Ardha Hanumanasana

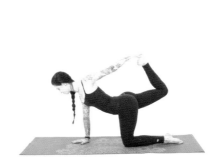

5   Vyaghrasana

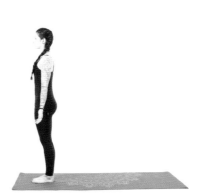

7   Sun Salutation B— see page 2

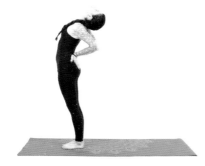

8   Tadasana

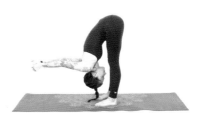

9   Yoga Mudrasana

10. *Alanasana* (High Lunge Pose)

11. *Parivrtta Alanasana* (Twisted High Lunge Pose)

12. *Utthan Pristhasana* (Lizard Pose)

13. Plank Pose

14. *Urdhva Mukha Svanasana* (Upward Facing Dog Pose). Hold for 5 cycles of breath.

15. *Balasana* (Child's Pose)

16. Repeat steps 10 through 15 on other side

17. *Ustrasana* (Camel Pose)

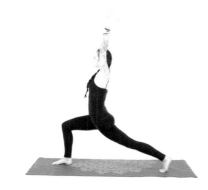

10 Alanasana

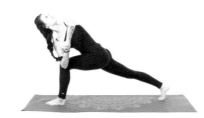

11 Parivrtta Alanasana

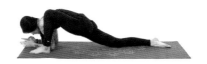

12 Utthan Pristhasana

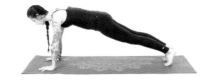

13 Plank

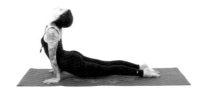

14 Urdhva Mukha Svanasana

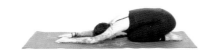

15 Balasana

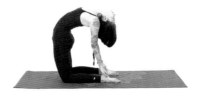

17 Ustrasana

Wheel Pose (Urdhva Dhanurasana)

When I taught yoga at Belle Sherman Elementary School in Ithaca, New York, Wheel Pose was the crowd favorite. Kids seem to love this pose. They drop back into it from standing, and fall down on their backs giggling when they decide they are done. For many of my students, it seems like somewhere in the transition from childhood to adulthood, the love affair has ended. I invite you to rekindle your love, develop a new crush, or sustain an old passion with this heart and hip opening sequence.

1. *Supta Baddha Konasana* (Reclined Bound Angle Pose)

2. *Setu Bandhasana* (Bridge Pose)

3. *Supta Virasana* (Reclined Hero Pose). Note: Come into the restorative version of this pose, using as many pillows as you like behind the back.

4. Cat/Cow in Table Top

5. *Anjaneyasana* (Knee Down Lunge)

6. *Ardha Hanumanasana* (Half Split Pose)

7. Flow between steps 5 and 6.

8. *Alanasana* (High Lunge Pose)

9. *Parivrtta Alanasana* (Revolved High Lunge Pose)

10. *Baddha Virabhadrasana* (Humble Warrior Pose)

Continued on page 88.

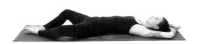

1   Supta Baddha Konasana

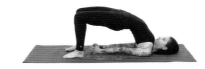

2   Setu Bandhasana

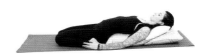

3   Supta Virasana

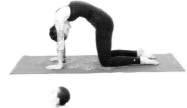

4   Cat/Cow in Table Top

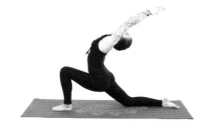

5   Anjaneyasana

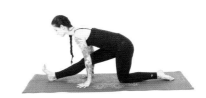

6   Ardha Hanumanasana

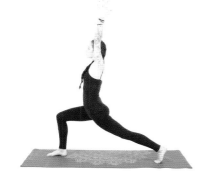

8   Alanasana

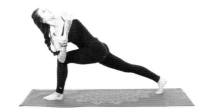

9   Parivrtta Alanasana

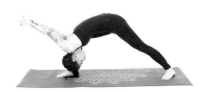

10   Baddha Virabhadrasana

11. *Virabhadrasana II* (Warrior II)

12. *Prasarita Padottanasana* (Standing Wide-Legged Forward Fold), with *Gomukhasana* (Cow Face Pose) bind in the arms, using a strap as you warm up.

13. Repeat steps 5 through 12 on other side.

14. *Surya Namaskar A* (Sun Salutation A—see page 1). Repeat 5 times.

15. *Bhujangasana* (Cobra Pose)

16. Sphinx Pose

17. *Balasana* (Child's Pose)

18. *Setu Bandhasana* (Bridge Pose)

19. *Urdhva Dhanurasana* (Wheel Pose)

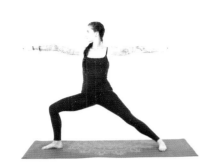

11 Virabhadrasana II

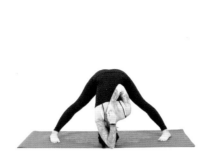

12 Prasarita Padottanasana
with Gomukhasana

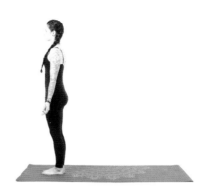

14 Sun Salutation A—
see page 1

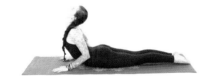

15 Bhujangasana

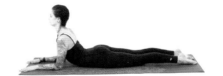

16 Sphinx

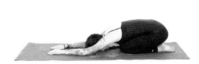

17 Balasana

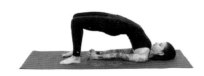

18 Setu Bandhasana

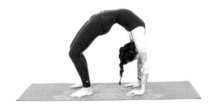

19 Urdhva Dhanurasana

Bound Balancing Half Moon Pose
(Ardha Chandra Chapasana)

Prepare for this pose from a Table Top position. Come into a knee-down variation of Balancing Half Moon. Take the grounded shin and foot off to the side like a kickstand for more support. From there, if you feel stable, create a bind by taking your hand to the foot or ankle that is extended over the ground. If it's out of your reach, continue to work toward this pose in the knee-down variation before attempting it from ARDHA CHANDRASANA (Balancing Half Moon).

1. URDHVA HASTASANA (Upward Hands Pose). Note: Stretch side to side here to lengthen the muscles around your ribs.

2. ADHO MUKHA SVANASANA (Downward Facing Dog Pose)

3. URDHVA MUKHA SVANASANA (Upward Facing Dog Pose)

4. Flow between steps 2 and 3 five times.

5. BALASANA (Child's Pose). Note: Walk the hands to the right side of your mat and then to the left, holding each for 5 cycles of breath.

6. Cat/Cow in Table Top

7. VIRABHADRASANA II (Warrior II)

8. VIPARITA VIRABHADRASANA (Peaceful Warrior Pose)

9. UTTHITA PARSVAKONASANA (Extended Side Angle Pose). Note: In this variation, take the top arm behind the lower back and try to grab the thigh of the bent leg.

10. Keeping the arm around the back, move into TRIKONASANA (Triangle Pose)

11. VIRABHADRASANA II (Warrior II)

12. Repeat steps 7 through 11 on other side.

13. BHUJANGASANA (Cobra Pose)

CONTINUED ON PAGE 92.

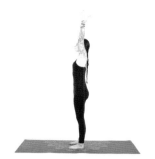

1 Urdhva
Hastasana

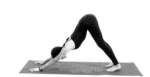

2 Adho Mukha
Svanasana

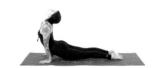

3 Urdhva Mukha
Svanasana

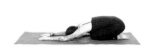

5 Balasana

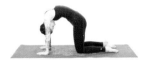
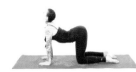

6 Cat/Cow in
Table Top

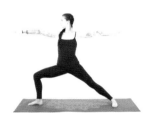

7 Virabhadrasana II

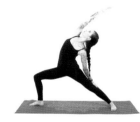

8 Viparita
Virabhadrasana

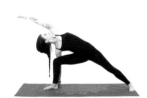

9 Utthita
Parsvakonasana

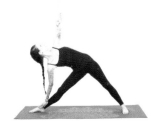

10 Trikonasana

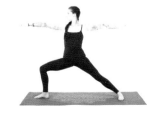

11 Virabhadrasana II

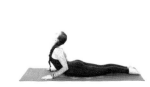

13 Bhujangasana

14. *Dhanurasana* (Bow Pose)

15. *Balasana* (Child's Pose)

16. *Paschimottanasna* (Seated Forward Fold)

17. *Anjaneyasana* (Knee Down Lunge)

18. *Ardha Hanumanasana* (Half Split)

19. *Alanasana* (High Lunge Pose)

20. *Natarajasana* (Dancer's Pose)

21. *Virabhadrasana II* (Warrior II)

22. *Trikonasana* (Triangle Pose)

23. *Ardha Chandrasana* (Balancing Half Moon Pose)

24. *Ardha Chandra Chapasana* (Bound Balancing Half Moon Pose)

25. Repeat steps 17 through 24 on other side.

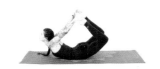

14 Dhanurasana

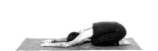

15 Balasana

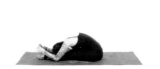

16 Paschimottanasana

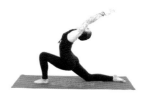

17 Anjaneyasana

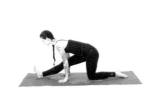

18 Ardha
Hanumanasana

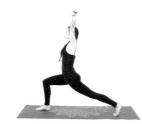

19 Alanasana

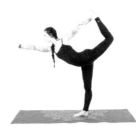

20 Natarajasana

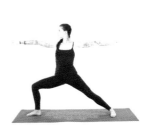

21 Virabhadrasana II

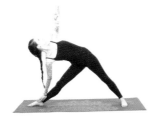

22 Trikonasana

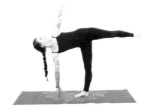

23 Ardha
Chandrasana

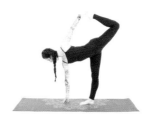

24 Ardha Chandra
Chapasana

Compass Pose (Parivrtta Surya Yantrasana)

Given this posture's name, it's ironic how easy it is to feel "lost" when you're first attempting the pose. My arm goes *WHERE?!* My leg is supposed to do *WHAT?!* Let the pose guide you: if your upper back is feeling constricted, emphasize shoulder openers; if your hamstrings refuse the leg extension, focus on the legs. With a lot of patience and a lot of breath, you'll find your way.

1. *Supta Padangusthasana* (Reclined Big Toe Pose)
2. *Supta Trivikramasana* (Reclined Vishnu Pose)
3. *Urdhva Mukha Paschimottanasana* (Upward Facing Forward Fold Pose)
4. Repeat steps 1 through 3 on other side.
5. *Tadasana* (Mountain Pose)
6. *Surya Namaskar A* (Sun Salutation A—see page 1). Repeat 5 times.
7. *Garudasana* (Eagle Pose)
8. *Virabhadrasana I* (Warrior I)
9. *Baddha Virabhadrasana* (Humble Warrior Pose)
10. *Virabhadrasana II* (Warrior II Pose)

Continued on page 96.

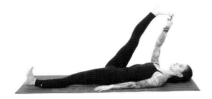

1 Supta Padangusthasana

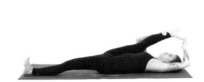

2 Supta Trivikramasana

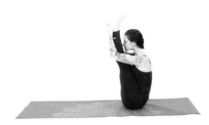

3 Urdhva Mukha Paschimottanasana

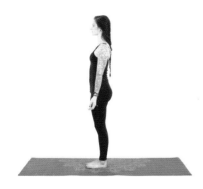

5 Tadasana

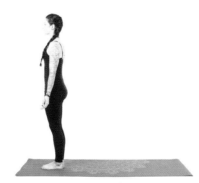

6 Sun Salutation A— see page 1

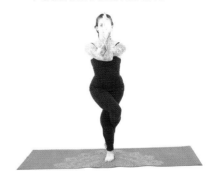

7 Garudasana

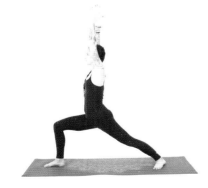

8 Virabhadrasana I

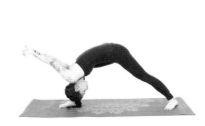

9 Baddha Virabhadrasana

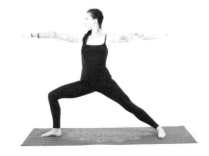

10 Virabhadrasana II

11. *Viparita Virabhadrasana* (Peaceful Warrior Pose)

12. *Trikonasana* (Triangle Pose)

13. *Virabhadrasana II* (Warrior II Pose)

14. Repeat steps 7 through 13 on other side.

15. *Salabhasana* (Locust Pose). Note: Take this pose twice, once with the arms reaching back, the second with the arms reaching forward.

16. *Balasana* (Child's Pose)

17. *Navasana* (Boat Pose). Note: Take this pose three times. The last time, take your pointer and middle fingers and grab the big toes, trying to straighten the legs with the toe bind.

18. *Ardha Matsyendrasana* (Half Seated Twist). Repeat on other side.

19. *Parivrtta Surya Yantrasana* (Compass Pose). Repeat on other side.

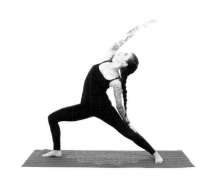

11 Viparita Virabhadrasana

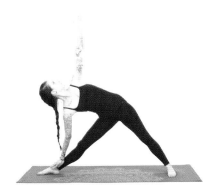

12 Trikonasana

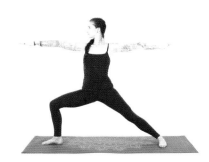

13 Virabhadrasana II

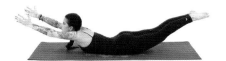

15 Salabhasana

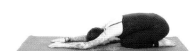

16 Balasana

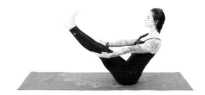

17 Navasana

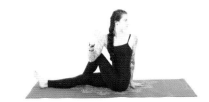

18 Ardha Matsyendrasana

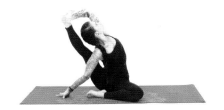

19 Parivrtta Surya Yantrasana

Half Frog Pose (Ardha Bhekasana)

The trick to a well-aligned *Ardha Bhekasana* (Half Frog Pose) is to keep the chest moving forward and the navel lifted. While focusing on the extreme flexion in the knee, it's easy to forget about the back and to collapse in the torso. Use the prep work in Sphinx to remember to roll the shoulders back, engage the core, and move the heart forward. You'll be leaping to frog in no time!

1. *Supta Virasana* (Reclined Hero Pose). Note: Come into the restorative version of this pose, using as many pillows as you like behind the back.

2. *Setu Bandhasana* (Bridge Pose)

3. Cat/Cow in Table Top

4. *Anjaneyasana* (Knee Down Lunge)

5. *Ardha Hanumanasana* (Half Split)

6. Flow between steps 4 and 5. Repeat on other side.

7. *Adho Mukha Svanasana* (Downward Facing Dog Pose). Note: Pedal the legs in place, bending one knee and then the other.

8. *Bhujangasana* (Cobra Pose)

9. Sphinx Pose. Hold for 1–2 minutes, focus on drawing the navel toward the spine.

Continued on page 100.

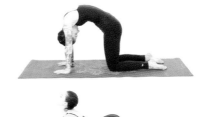

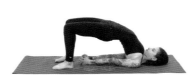

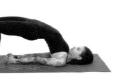

1 Supta Virasana

2 Setu Bandhasana

3 Cat/Cow in Table Top

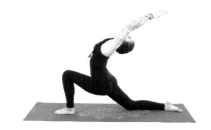

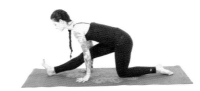

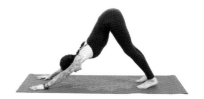

4 Anjaneyasana

5 Ardha Hanumanasana

7 Adho Mukha Svanasana

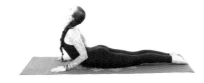

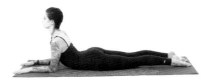

8 Bhujangasana

9 Sphinx

10. *Balasana* (Child's Pose)

11. *Virasana* (Hero Pose), with *Garudasana* (Eagle Pose) arms. Draw circles with elbows in both directions. Repeat with opposite arm on top.

12. *Adho Mukha Svanasana* (Downward Facing Dog Pose)

13. *Urdhva Mukha Svanasana* (Upward Facing Dog Pose)

14. Flow between steps 12 and 13 five times, holding each *Urdhva Mukha Svanasana* for 3 cycles of breath.

15. *Balasana* (Child's Pose)

16. *Ardha Bhekasana* (Half Frog Pose). Repeat on other side.

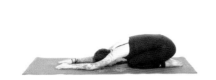

10 Balasana

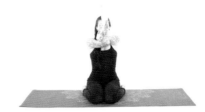

11 Virasana with
Garudasana arms

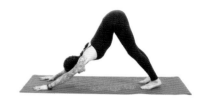

12 Adho Mukha
Svanasana

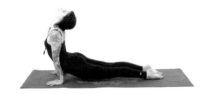

13 Urdhva Mukha Svanasana

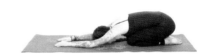

15 Balasana

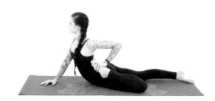

16 Ardha Bhekasana

One-Footed King Pigeon Pose
(Eka Pada Rajakapotasana)

Once, I was taking a friend's yoga class and she said, "Do not let the beauty of the pose overcome the wisdom of the body." This is an incredibly beautiful pose, but I caution against forcing your body into it at the expense of your lower back. If you have any back injury or very tight hips, take the variation where you reach one arm back for the ankle or foot (and/or use a strap). Find the internal beauty in the experience.

1. *Supta Baddha Konasana* (Reclined Bound Angle Pose)
2. *Setu Bandhasana* (Bridge Pose)
3. *Gomukhasana* (Cow Face Pose). Repeat on other side.
4. Cat/Cow in Table Top
5. *Surya Namaskar A* (Sun Salutation A—see page 1). Repeat 5 times.
6. *Surya Namaskar B* (Sun Salutation B—see page 2). Repeat 5 times.
7. *Vrkasana* (Tree Pose). Repeat on other side.
8. *Anjaneyasana* (Knee Down Lunge)
9. *Parivrtta Alanasana* (Revolved High Lunge)
10. Step forward to *Parivrtta Utkatasana* (Revolved Chair Pose)

CONTINUED ON PAGE 104.

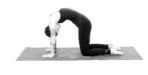

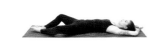

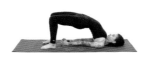

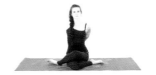

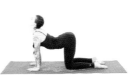

1 Supta Baddha Konasana

2 Setu Bandhasana

3 Gomukhasana

4 Cat/Cow in Table Top

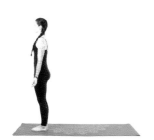

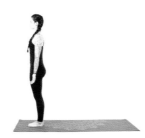

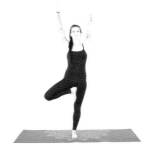

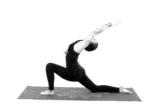

5 Sun Salutation A— see page 1

6 Sun Salutation B— see page 2

7 Vrksasana

8 Anjaneyasana

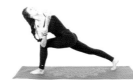

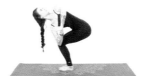

9 Parivrtta Alanasana

10 Parivrtta Utkatasana

11. *Natarajasana* (Dancer's Pose)

12. *Vinyasa* to repeat steps 8 through 11 on other side.

13. *Virabhadrasana II* (Warrior II)

14. *Utthita Parsvakonasana* (Extended Side Angle Pose)

15. *Trikonasana* (Triangle Pose)

16. Repeat steps 13 through 15 on other side.

17. *Bhujangasana* (Cobra Pose)

18. *Dhanurasana* (Bow Pose)

19. *Balasana* (Child's Pose). Note: Walk the hands to the right side of your mat and then to the left, holding each for 5 cycles of breath.

20. *Supta Eka Pada Rajakapotasana* (Resting Pigeon Pose)

21. *Eka Pada Rajakapotasana* (One Footed King Pigeon Pose)

22. Repeat steps 20 and 21 on other side.

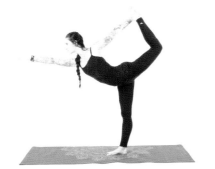

11 Natarajasana

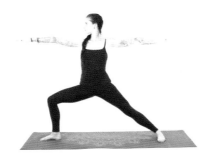

13 Virabhadrasana II

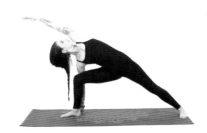

14 Utthita Parsvakonasana

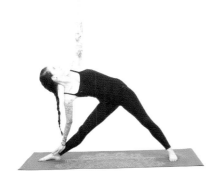

15 Trikonasana

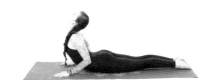

17 Bhujangasana

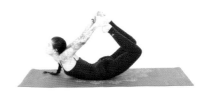

18 Dhanurasana

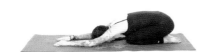

19 Balasana

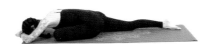

20 Supta Eka Pada
Rajakapotasana

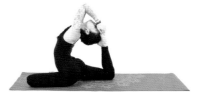

21 Eka Pada Rajakapotasana

Pigeon Pose (Kapotasana)

Anybody out there as surprised as me to find out what the full version of Pigeon Pose actually looks like? Turns out this incredibly deep quad stretch and heart opener has more in common with Wheel Pose (*Urdhva Dhanurasana*) and Camel Pose (*Ustrasana*) than with the "Pigeon Pose" you often hear about in yoga classes. The other "Pigeon Pose" is actually a variation of *Eka Pada Rajakapotasana* (One-Footed King Pigeon Pose) and, frankly, a whole 'nother can of worms. For a longer sequence, combine the flow from *Eka Pada Rajakapotasana* with this sequence, including overlapping poses, and get an amazing warm-up for an amazing posture!

1. *Supta Virasana* (Reclined Hero Pose). Note: Come into the restorative version of this pose, using as many pillows as you like behind the back.

2. *Supta Matsyendrasana* (Supine Twist Pose). Repeat on other side.

3. *Setu Bandhasana* (Bridge Pose)

4. Cat/Cow in Table Top

5. *Gomukhasana* (Cow Face Pose). Repeat on other side.

6. *Anjaneyasana* (Knee Down Lunge)

7. *Ardha Hanumanasana* (Half Split Pose)

8. Flow between steps 6 and 7.

9. *Alanasana* (High Lunge Pose)

10. *Parivrtta Alanasana* (Revolved High Lunge Pose)

11. *Baddha Virabhadrasana* (Humble Warrior Pose)

12. *Virabhadrasana I* (Warrior I)

CONTINUED ON PAGE 108.

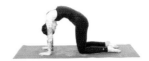

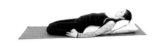

1　Supta Virasana

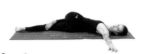

2　Supta Matsyendrasana

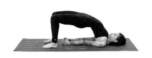

3　Setu Bandhasana

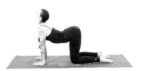

4　Cat/Cow in Table Top

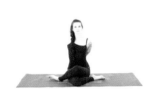

5　Gomukhasana

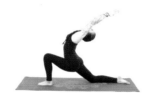

6　Anjaneyasana

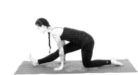

7　Ardha Hanumanasana

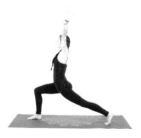

9　Alanasana

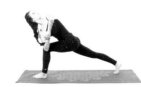

10　Parivrtta Alanasana

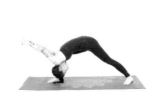

11　Baddha Virabhadrasana

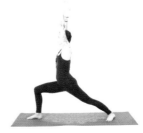

12　Virabhadrasana I

13. Repeat steps 6 through 12 on other side.

14. *Surya Namaskar A* (Sun Salutation A—see page 1). Repeat 5 times.

15. *Surya Namaskar B* (Sun Salutation B—see page 2). Repeat 5 times.

16. *Bhujangasana* (Cobra Pose)

17. *Dhanurasana* (Bow Pose)

18. *Balasana* (Child's Pose)

19. *Urdhva Dhanurasana* (Wheel Pose)

20. *Ustrasana* (Camel Pose)

21. *Balasana* (Child's Pose)

22. *Kapotasana* (Pigeon Pose)

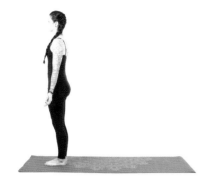

14 Sun Salutation A—see page 1

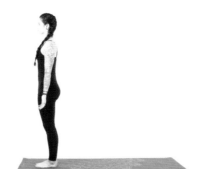

15 Sun Salutation B— see page 2

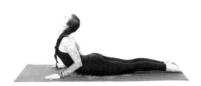

16 Bhujangasana

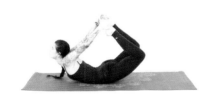

17 Dhanurasana

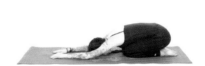

18 Balasana

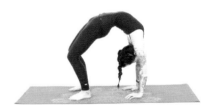

19 Urdhva Dhanurasana

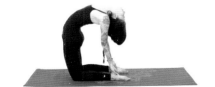

20 Ustrasana

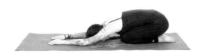

21 Balasana

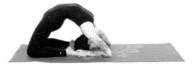

22 Kapotasana

Create New Perspectives

Inversions

Half Bound Standing Lotus Forward Fold
(*Ardha Baddha Padmottanasana*)

In the Ashtanga Yoga Primary series, this pose shows up surprisingly early. It requires a significant amount of knee flexion, hamstring stretch, and shoulder opening. If you have any knee injuries, put your ankle to your knee before coming into the forward fold instead of bringing your foot to the hip crease.

1. *VAJRASANA* (Diamond Pose)

2. *USTRASANA* (Camel Pose). Note: Keep the hands on the sacrum (above the tailbone) while you warm up.

3. *PASCHIMOTTANASANA* (Seated Forward Fold)

4. *JANU SIRSASANA* (Head to Knee Pose)

5. *SUPTA EKA PADA RAJAKAPOTASANA* (Resting Pigeon Pose). Come into this pose by swinging the straight leg in *JANU SIRSASANA* behind you and bowing over the bent knee.

6. *GOMUKHASANA* (Cow Face Pose). Come into this pose by (carefully) swinging the leg behind you forward again, crossing it over the bent knee.

7. *BADDHA KONASANA* (Bound Angle Pose)

8. Repeat steps 4 through 6 on other side.

CONTINUED ON PAGE 114.

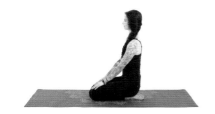

1 Vajrasana

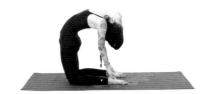

2 Ustrasana

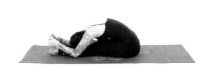

3 Paschimottanasana

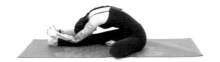

4 Janu Sirsasana

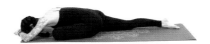

5 Supta Eka Pada
   Rajakapotasana

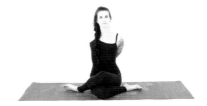

6 Gomukhasana

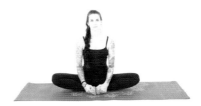

7 Baddha Konasana

9. *Adho Mukha Svanasana* (Downward Facing Dog Pose). Note: Take some time to pedal the heels in place.

10. *Uttanasana* (Standing Forward Fold)

11. *Yoga Mudrasana, variation* (Standing Forward Fold with Hands Interlaced Behind Back)

12. *Utthita Pavana Muktasana* (Standing Wind Relieving Pose). Repeat other side.

13. *Vrksasana* (Tree Pose). Repeat other side.

14. *Natarajasana* (Dancer's Pose). Repeat other side.

15. *Ardha Baddha Padmottanasana* (Half Bound Standing Lotus Forward Fold). Repeat other side.

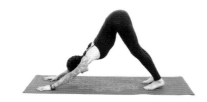

9 Adho Mukha Svanasana

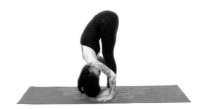

10 Uttanasana

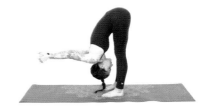

11 Yoga Mudrasana

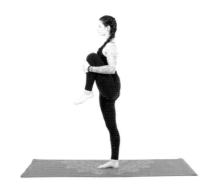

12 Utthita Pavana Muktasana

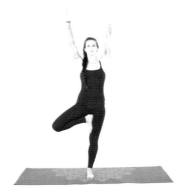

13 Vrksasana

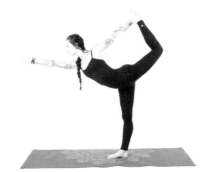

14 Natarajasana

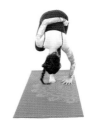

15 Ardha Baddha
Padmottanasana

Standing Splits (Urdhva Prasarita Eka Padasana)

This is another one of my favorite poses to practice against a wall. Come into a Downward Facing Dog with your heels to the wall. Take your right thigh into your chest, point your toes, and then extend the leg against the wall, with the top of the foot pressing into the wall. From there, walk your hands toward the left foot until you find an intense (but manageable) stretch. Hold for 5 cycles of breath and then repeat with the left leg after a break in Child's Pose.

1. *Supta Padangusthasana* (Reclined Big Toe Pose). Repeat on other side.

2. *Urdhva Mukha Paschimottanasana* (Upward Facing Forward Fold Pose)

3. *Navasana* (Boat Pose)

4. *Ardha Matsyendrasana* (Half Seated Twist). Repeat on other side.

5. *Navasana* (Boat Pose)

6. Reverse Table Top

7. *Navasana* (Boat Pose)

8. *Purvottanasana* (Reverse Plank Pose)

9. Cat/Cow in Table Top

Continued on page 118.

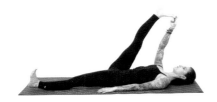

1 Supta Padangusthasana

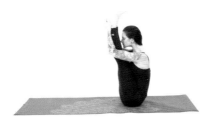

2 Urdhva Mukha
Paschimottanasana

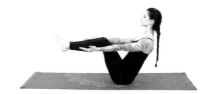

3 Navasana

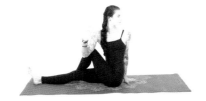

4 Ardha Matsyendrasana

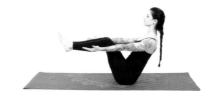

5 Navasana

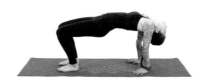

6 Reverse Table Top

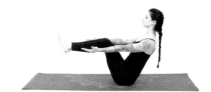

7 Navasana

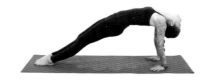

8 Purvottanasana

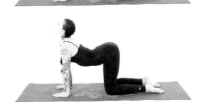

9 Cat/Cow in Table Top

10. *Uttanasana* (Standing Forward Fold). Note: Hold for 1–2 minutes, at first bending and straightening knees in the pose and then finding stillness.

11. *Surya Namaskar A* (Sun Salutation A—see page 1). Repeat 5 times.

12. *Anjaneyasana* (Knee Down Lunge)

13. *Ardha Hanumanasana* (Half Split Pose)

14. *Alanasana* (High Lunge Pose)

15. *Prasarita Padottanasana* (Standing Wide-Legged Forward Fold)

16. *Parsvottanasana* (Pyramid Pose)

17. *Virabhadrasana III* (Warrior III Pose)

18. *Urdhva Prasarita Eka Padasana* (Standing Splits)

19. Repeat steps 12 through 18 on other side.

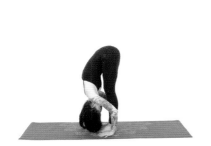

10 Uttanasana

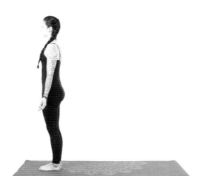

11 Sun Salutation A—see page 1

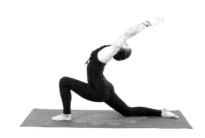

12 Anjaneyasana

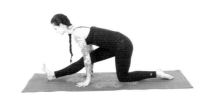

13 Ardha Hanumanasana

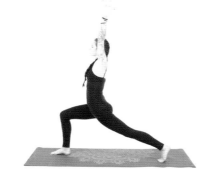

14 Alanasana

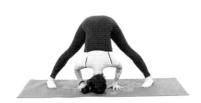

15 Prasarita Padottanasana

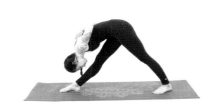

16 Parsvottanasana

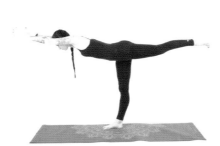

17 Virabhadrasana III

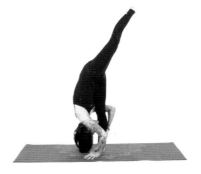

18 Urdhva Prasarita Eka Padasana

Supported Shoulder Stand (Salamba Sarvangasana)

The "peak pose" of this sequence is Supported Shoulder Stand. This pose, combined in succession with the peak poses of the next two sequences (Plow Pose and Ear Pressure Pose), will be familiar to practioners of Ashtanga yoga. In that style of yoga, these three poses are taught at the end of every single class in preparation for Savasana. While many yoga studios do not use props during Shoulder Stand, I personally advocate for placing one to three blankets underneath your shoulders and resting your head on the floor. This protects the cervical spine and helps prevent injury.

1. *SUKHASANA* (Easy Seat). Note: Enjoy gentle head and neck rolls, pausing and breathing into any stretch you find.

2. *SASANGASANA* (Rabbit Pose)

3. *ANAHATASANA* (Extended Puppy Pose)

4. Cat/Cow in Table Top

5. *PASCHIMOTTANASANA* (Seated Forward Fold)

6. *ARDHA MATYSENDRASANA* (Half Seated Twist). Repeat on other side.

7. *ADHO MUKHA SVANASANA* (Downward Facing Dog Pose)

8. *YOGA MUDRASANA, VARIATION* (Standing Forward Fold with Hands Interlaced Behind Back)

9. *SETU BANDHASANA* (Bridge Pose). Note: Do this pose twice. The first time, reach the hands toward the heels alongside the torso. The second time, interlace the hands below the lower back.

10. *HALASANA* (Plow Pose)

11. *SALAMBA SARVANGASANA* (Supported Shoulderstand)

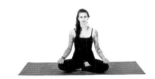

1   Sukhasana

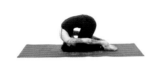

2   Sasangasana

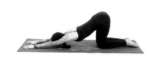

3   Anahatasana

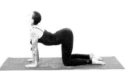

4   Cat/Cow in Table Top

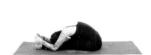

5   Paschimottanasana

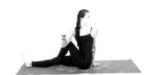

6   Ardha Matsyendrasana

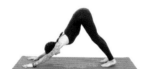

7   Adho Mukha Svanasana

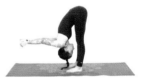

8   Yoga Mudrasana

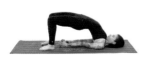

9   Setu Bandhasana

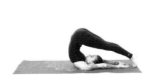

10   Halasana

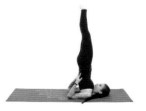

11   Salamba Sarvangasana

Plow Pose (Halasana)

From Shoulder Stand Pose (*Salamba Sarvangasana*), the feet lower to the floor above the head. As you are beginning to practice this pose, there's a good chance the feet will not be able to make it all the way to the ground. While you can definitely use props to help you on your way, I have modified the warm-up sequence for Shoulder Stand Pose to include a few extra stretches to help you on the way to a deeper Plow Pose.

1. *Supta Padangusthasana* (Reclined Big Toe Pose). Repeat on other side.
2. *Urdhva Mukha Paschimottanasana* (Upward Facing Forward Fold Pose)
3. *Paschimottanasana* (Seated Forward Fold)
4. Cat/Cow in Table Top
5. *Sasangasana* (Rabbit Pose)
6. *Anahatasanana* (Extended Puppy Pose)
7. *Gomukhasana* (Cow Face Pose). Repeat on other side.
8. *Ardha Matysendrasana* (Half Seated Twist). Repeat on other side.
9. *Adho Mukha Svanasana* (Downward Facing Dog Pose)

Continued on page 124.

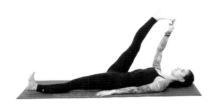

1 Supta Padangusthasana

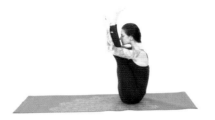

2 Urdhva Mukha
Paschimottanasana

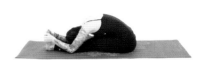

3 Paschimottanasana

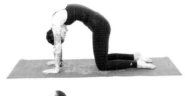

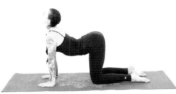

4 Cat/Cow in Table Top

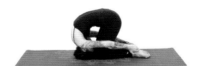

5 Sasangasana

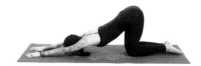

6 Anahatasana

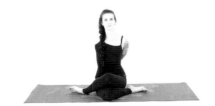

7 Gomukhasana

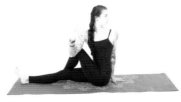

8 Ardha Matsyendrasana

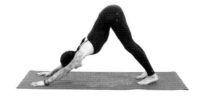

9 Adho Mukha Svanasana

10. *Baddha Virabhadrasana* (Humble Warrior Pose)

11. *Alanasana* (High Lunge Pose)

12. *Parivrtta Alanasana* (Revolved High Lunge Pose)

13. *Parivrtta Utkatasana* (Revolved Chair Pose)

14. *Uttanasana* (Standing Forward Fold)

15. *Vinyasa* to repeat steps 9 through 14 on other side.

16. *Yoga Mudrasana, variation* (Standing Forward Fold with Hands Interlaced Behind Back)

17. *Setu Bandhasana* (Bridge Pose). Note: Do this pose twice. The first time, reach the hands toward the heels alongside the torso. The second time, take the hands to the lower back to prep for *Salamba Sarvangasana*.

18. *Salamba Sarvangasana* (Supported Shoulderstand)

19. *Halasana* (Plow Pose)

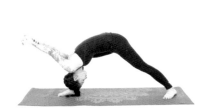

10 Baddha Virabhadrasana

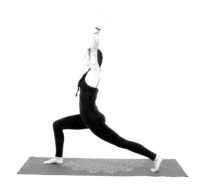

11 Alanasana

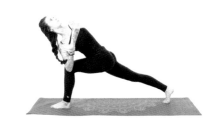

12 Parivrtta Alanasana

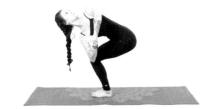

13 Parivrtta Utkatasana

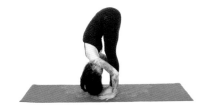

14 Uttanasana

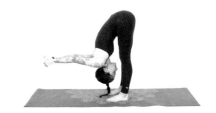

16 Yoga Mudrasana

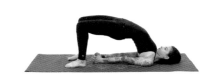

17 Setu Bandhasana

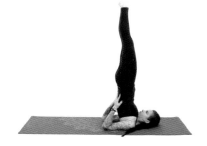

18 Salamba Sarvangasana

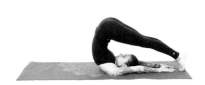

19 Halasana

Ear Pressure Pose (*Karnapidasana*)

In my first book, *The Joy of Yoga*, I included a sequence of poses titled "Yoga Poses That Are Awkward to Do Naked." In my humble(ish) opinion, Ear Pressure Pose is the peak pose of that particular sequence. You're welcome to practice this sequence wearing whatever clothing (or lack thereof) that you fancy—just don't send pictures.

1. *Supta Baddha Konasana* (Reclined Bound Angle Pose)
2. *Ananda Balasana* (Happy Baby Pose)
3. *Malasana* (Seated Squat Pose)
4. Cat/Cow in Table Top
5. *Sukhasana* (Easy Seat). Note: Enjoy gentle head and neck rolls, pausing and breathing into any stretch you find.
6. *Simhasana Pranayama* (Lion's Breath) in *Sukhasana* (Easy Seat)
7. *Sasangasana* (Rabbit Pose)
8. *Anahatasana* (Extended Puppy Pose) Note: "Thread the Needle" in this pose, taking one arm underneath the other. Repeat on other side.
9. *Uttanasana* (Standing Forward Fold)

Continued on page 128.

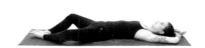
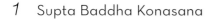

1   Supta Baddha Konasana

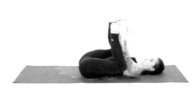

2   Ananda Balasana

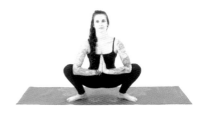

3   Malasana

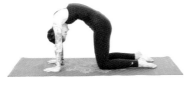
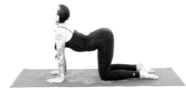

4   Cat/Cow in Table Top

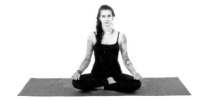

5   Sukhasana

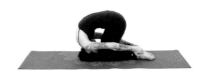

7   Sasangasana

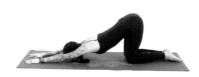

8   Anahatasana

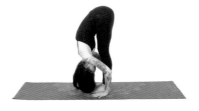

9   Uttanasana

10. *Adho Mukha Svanasana* (Downward Facing Dog Pose)

11. *Baddha Virabhadrasana* (Humble Warrior Pose)

12. *Prasarita Padottanasana* (Standing Wide-Legged Forward Fold), with *Gomukhasana* (Cow Face Pose) bind in the arms.

13. *Parsvottanasana* (Pyramid Pose)

14. Repeat steps 10 through 13 on other side.

15. *Yoga Mudrasana, variation* (Standing Forward Fold with Hands Interlaced Behind Back)

16. *Setu Bandhasana* (Bridge Pose)

17. *Salamba Sarvangasana* (Supported Shoulderstand)

18. *Halasana* (Plow Pose)

19. *Karnapidasana* (Ear Pressure Pose)

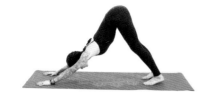

10 Adho Mukha
Svanasana

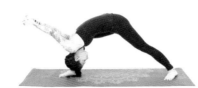

11 Baddha
Virabhadrasana

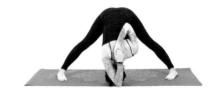

12 Prasarita Padottanasana
with Gomukhasana

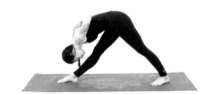

13 Parsvottanasana

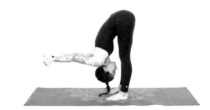

15 Yoga Mudrasana

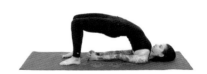

16 Setu Bandhasana

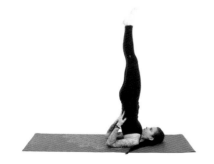

17 Salamba
Sarvangasana

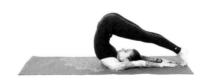

18 Halasana

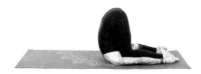

19 Karnapidasana

Supported Headstand (*Salamba Sirsasana*)

Going upside down can be disorienting. If we aren't used to it, our proprioceptive sense (an awareness of our body's position in space, gained from information from the inner ear and stretch receptors) might sound a red alarm. To help prepare the mind for Headstand, even more so than the body, take some time in standing inversions and feel the ground safely underneath you. Then move onto standing balancing poses to get more accustomed to feeling unsteady, knowing that you are safe.

1. *Tadasana* (Mountain Pose) Note: Close the eyes and notice the weight shift in the feet.

2. *Uttanasana* (Standing Forward Fold)

3. *Yoga Mudrasana, variation* (Standing Forward Fold with Hands Interlaced Behind Back)

4. *Adho Mukha Svanasana* (Downward Facing Dog Pose)

5. Dolphin Pose

6. *Vrksasana* (Tree Pose). Repeat on other side.

7. *Utthita Pavana Muktasana* (Standing Knee into Chest Pose). Repeat on other side.

Continued on page 132.

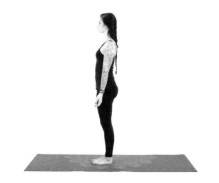

1 Tadasana

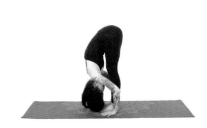

2 Uttanasana

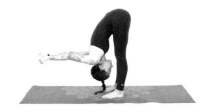

3 Yoga Mudrasana

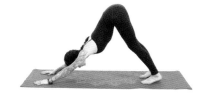

4 Adho Mukha Svanasana

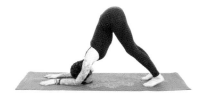

5 Dolphin

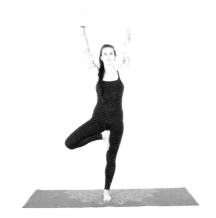

6 Vrksasana

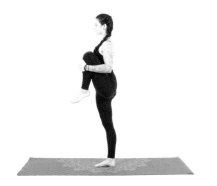

7 Utthita Pavana Muktasana

8. *NATARAJASANA* (Dancer's Pose). Repeat on other side.

9. Cat/Cow in Table Top

10. *SASANGASANA* (Rabbit Pose)

11. *ANAHATASANA* (Extended Puppy Pose)

12. *BALASANA* (Child's Pose)

13. *SALAMBA SIRSASANA* (Supported Headstand)

14. *BALASANA* (Child's Pose)

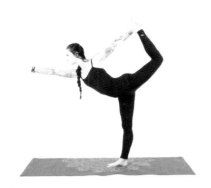

8 Natarajasana

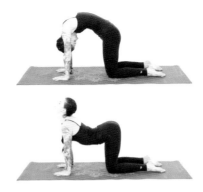

9 Cat/Cow in Table Top

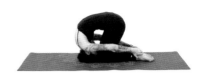

10 Sasangasana

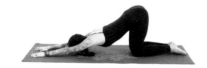

11 Anahatasana

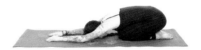

12 Balasana

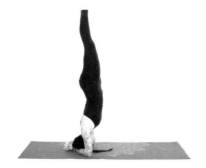

13 Salamba Sirsasana

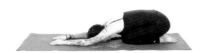

14 Balasana

Tripod Headstand (Salamba Sirsasana II)

Here's an exciting way to incorporate Tripod Headstand into your yoga practice: after you feel comfortable in the pose, start to come into it when you're in a Standing Wide-Legged Forward Fold (*PRASARITA PADOTTANASANA*). Just don't try this in a packed class before you feel steady; no one wants to see yogis coming down like a row of dominoes.

1. Cat/Cow in Table Top
2. *SASANGASANA* (Rabbit Pose)
3. *ANAHATASANA* (Extended Puppy Pose)
4. Plank Pose
5. *CHATURANGA DANDASANA* (Four-Limbed Staff Pose). Note: This is the same arm position you'll be engaging in Tripod Headstand (*SALAMBA SIRSASANA II*).
6. *URDHVA MUKHA SVANASANA* (Upward Facing Dog Pose)
7. *ADHO MUKHA SVANASANA* (Downward Facing Dog Pose)
8. Repeat steps 4 through 7 five times.
9. Dolphin Pose
10. *BALASANA* (Child's Pose)
11. *PRASARITA PADOTTANASANA* (Standing Wide-Legged Forward Fold)
12. *BAKASANA* (Crow Pose). Note: Place a block in front of you in crow. With control, lightly place the crown of your head on the block and tuck your heels toward your seat. Inhale to lift back into Crow Pose.
13. *SALAMBA SIRSASANA II* (Tripod Headstand)

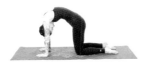

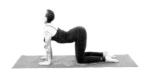

1 Cat/Cow in
Table Top

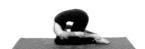

2 Sasangasana

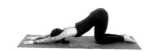

3 Anahatasana

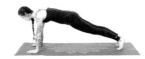

4 Plank

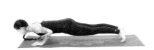

5 Chaturanga
Dandasana

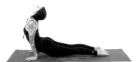

6 Urdhva Mukha
Svanasana

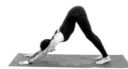

7 Adho Mukha
Svanasana

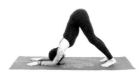

9 Dolphin

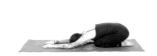

10 Balasana

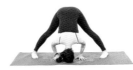

11 Prasarita
Padottanasana

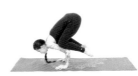

12 Bakasana

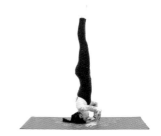

13 Salamba
Sirsasana II

Forearm Stand (*Pincha Mayurasana*)

I have fallen, ungracefully, out of Forearm Stand and have lived to tell the tale. I think this is one of the scariest inversions to practice away from a wall. In Headstand, I can tuck and roll out like a yogi ninja. In Handstand, I have the full use of my arms to pivot and spin out of a fall. In Forearm Stand . . . I eat dirt (see: "Arm Balancing Poses"). And while it isn't particularly pleasant, I'm okay. A few clunky falls also put me on the fast track to learning how to quickly press up from one forearm to a hand for the mobility necessary to cartwheel out.

1. *Gomukhasana* (Cow Face Pose). Use a strap in this posture until shoulders are warm. Repeat on other side.
2. Cat/Cow in Table Top
3. *Navasana* (Boat Pose). Repeat 3 times to warm up abdominal muscles.
4. Forearm Plank Pose
5. Dolphin Pose
6. Move forward and backward between steps 4 and 5.
7. *Balasana* (Child's Pose)

Continued on page 138.

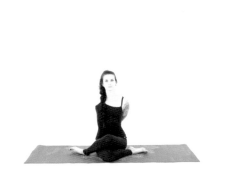

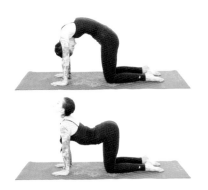

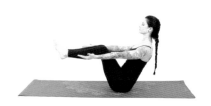

1   Gomukhasana

2   Cat/Cow in Table Top

3   Navasana

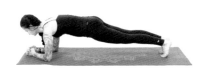

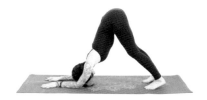

4   Forearm Plank

5   Dolphin

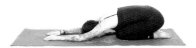

7   Balasana

8. *Surya Namaskar A* (Sun Salutation A—see page 1). Repeat 5 times.

9. *Parsvottanasana* (Pyramid Pose)

10. *Virabhadrasana III* (Warrior III Pose)

11. *Urdhva Prasarita Eka Padasana* (Standing Splits)

12. *Uttanasana* (Standing Forward Fold)

13. Repeat steps 9 through 12 on other side.

14. *Garudasana* (Eagle Pose). Repeat on other side.

15. Dolphin Pose

16. *Pincha Mayurasana* (Forearm Stand)

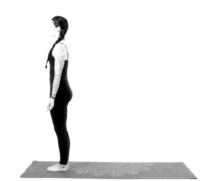

8 Sun Salutation
   A—see page 1

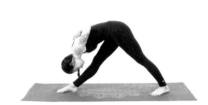

9 Parsvottanasana

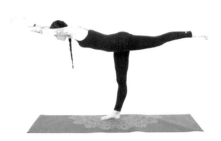

10 Virabhadrasana III

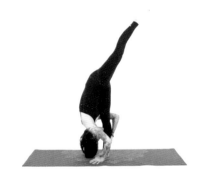

11 Urdhva Prasarita
    Eka Padasana

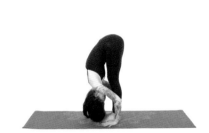

12 Uttanasana

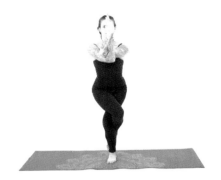

14 Garudasana

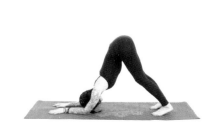

15 Dolphin

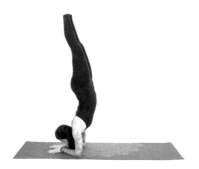

16 Pincha Mayurasana

Scorpion Pose in Forearm Balance
(Vrschikasana in Pincha Mayurasana)

Scorpion Pose in Forearm Balance combines the challenge of arm balances with the heart opening of deep back bends. In this sequence, we integrate the postures that develop stability in the shoulder girdle with postures that reduce tension in the upper back muscles. Try this pose using a wall; you'll get all of the benefits while developing balance.

1. *VIRASANA* (Hero Pose), with *GARUDASANA* (Eagle Pose) arms. Draw circles with elbows in both directions. Repeat with opposite arm on top.

2. Cat/Cow in Table Top

3. *NAVASANA* (Boat Pose). Repeat 3 times to warm up abdominal muscles.

4. Forearm Plank Pose

5. Dolphin Pose

6. Move forward and backward between steps 4 and 5.

7. *BALASANA* (Child's Pose)

8. *SURYA NAMASKAR A* (Sun Salutation A—see page 1). Repeat 5 times.

9. *SURYA NAMASKAR B* (Sun Salutation B—see page 2). Repeat 5 times.

CONTINUED ON PAGE 142.

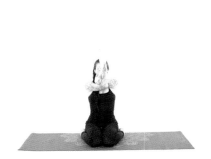

1 Virasana with Garudasana arms

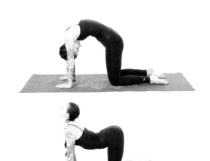

2 Cat/Cow in Table Top

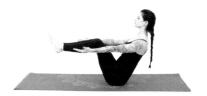

3 Navasana

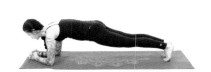

4 Forearm Plank

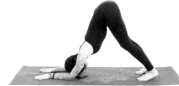

5 Dolphin

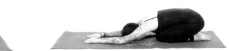

7 Balasana

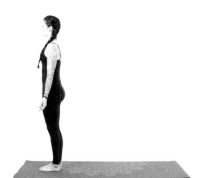

8 Sun Salutation A—see page 1

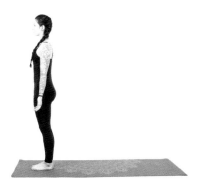

9 Sun Salutation B—see page 2

10. *Yoga Mudrasana, variation* (Standing Forward Fold with Hands Interlaced Behind Back)

11. Dolphin Pose

12. *Anahatasana* (Extended Puppy Pose)

13. *Parighasana* (Gate Pose). Repeat on other side.

14. *Ustrasana* (Camel Pose)

15. *Prasarita Padottanasana* (Standing Wide-Legged Forward Fold), with *Gomukhasana* (Cow Face Pose) bind in the arms. Repeat with opposite arm on top.

16. *Pincha Mayurasana* (Forearm Stand)

17. *Vrschikasana in Pincha Mayurasana* (Scorpion Pose in Forearm Balance)

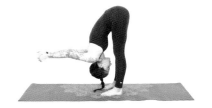

10 Yoga Mudrasana

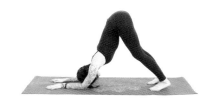

11 Dolphin

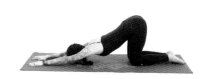

12 Anahatasana

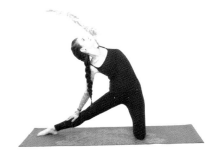

13 Parighasana

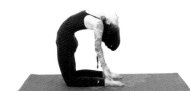

14 Ustrasana

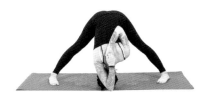

15 Prasarita Padottanasana with Gomukhasana

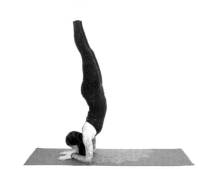

16 Pincha Mayurasana

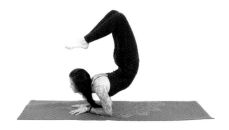

17 Vrschikasana in Pincha Mayurasana

Handstand Pose (*Adho Mukha Vrksasana*)

Yogi confession time: I cannot do a handstand (yet). I can kick up into one against a wall, but if you put me in the center of a room, I can't hold myself in the posture. I have been trying for years; when I first started trying, I couldn't kick up to the wall and would swing my legs through the air without any success. With that perspective, I've since made vast improvements to the pose and it's been a ton of fun to keep trying! There are whole workshops devoted to the art of Handstands, but here's a sequence to play around with at home while you put in your own practice time.

1. *VIRASANA* (Hero Pose), with *GARUDASANA* (Eagle Pose) arms. Draw circles with elbows in both directions. Repeat with opposite arm on top.
2. Cat/Cow in Table Top
3. Plank Pose. Hold for 1–2 minutes.
4. Forearm Plank Pose. Hold for 1–2 minutes.
5. *ANAHATASANA* (Extended Puppy Pose)
6. *UTTANASANA* (Standing Forward Fold). Hold for 1–2 minutes.
7. *SURYA NAMASKAR A* (Sun Salutation A—see page 1). Repeat 5 times.
8. *SURYA NAMASKAR B* (Sun Salutation B—see page 2). Repeat 5 times.
9. *URDHVA HASTASANA* (Upward Hands Pose) Note: Add lots of yummy side stretches!
10. *VRKSASANA* (Tree Pose)

CONTINUED ON PAGE 146.

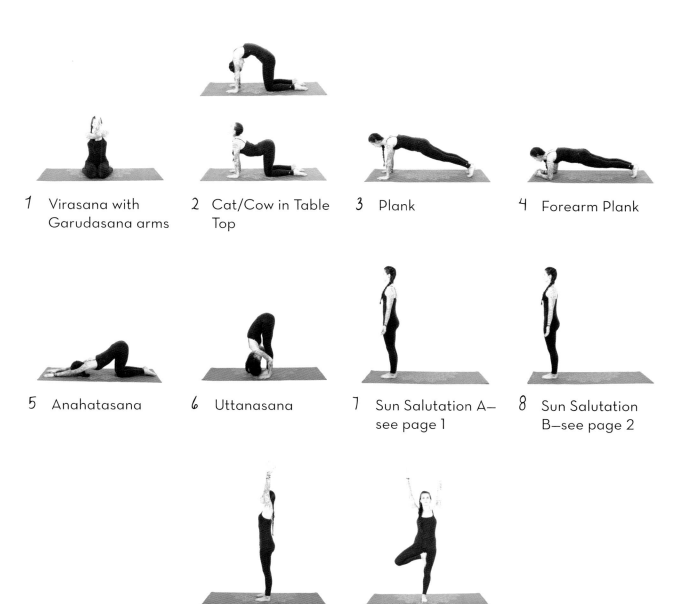

1 Virasana with Garudasana arms

2 Cat/Cow in Table Top

3 Plank

4 Forearm Plank

5 Anahatasana

6 Uttanasana

7 Sun Salutation A—see page 1

8 Sun Salutation B—see page 2

9 Urdhva Hastasana

10 Vrksasana

11. *Parsvottanasana* (Pyramid Pose)

12. *Virabhadrasana III* (Warrior III Pose)

13. *Urdhva Prasarita Eka Padasana* (Standing Splits)

14. *Malasana* (Seated Squat Pose)

15. *Vinyasa* to repeat steps 10 through 14 on other side.

16. *Bakasana* (Crow Pose)

17. *Prasarita Padottanasana* (Standing Wide-Legged Forward Fold), with *Gomukhasana* (Cow Face Pose) bind in the arms. Repeat with opposite arm on top.

18. *Salamba Sirsasana* (Supported Headstand Pose)

19. *Balasana* (Child's Pose)

20. *Adho Mukha Vrksasana* (Handstand Pose)

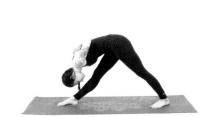

11 Parsvottanasana

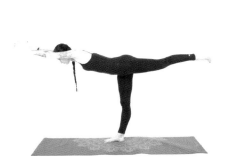

12 Virabhadrasana III

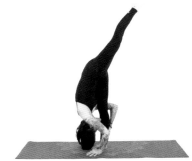

13 Urdhva Prasarita Eka Padasana

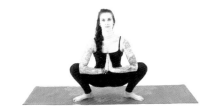

14 Malasana

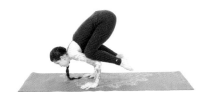

16 Bakasana

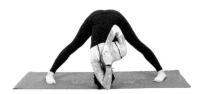

17 Prasarita Padottanasana with Gomukhasana

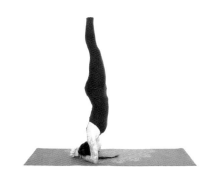

18 Salamba Sirsasana

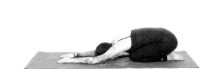

19 Balasana

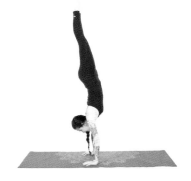

20 Adho Mukha Vrksasana

Melt Stress

Seated Floor Poses

Garland Pose (Malasana)

This is an incredible pose. Whenever I teach it and look around the room, it always appears as though half the room is in some particularly dreadful circle of Dante's INFERNO, while the other half the room wonders where they are supposed to feel a stretch. I understand this. A fair portion of the world spends its days in some variation of this pose, whether at work or at home—humans, to a certain degree, have the natural physical structure to rest in this pose. That said, there's another swath of humanity that sit in a chair all day and to whom this pose seems very, very unnatural. If you struggle in Garland Pose (sometimes called "Seated Squat"), then follow this sequence to open your hips and legs and—maybe—find comfort in it.

1. *Supta Baddha Konasana* (Reclined Bound Angle). Hold for 1–3 minutes.
2. *Supta Matsyendrasana* (Supine Twist Pose). Repeat on other side.
3. *Supta Pavana Muktasana* (Reclined Wind Relieving Pose). Note: Draw the knee out to the side for Supine Tree Pose and then repeat on other side.
4. *Apanasana* (Knees to Chest on Back)
5. *Balasana* (Child's Pose)
6. *Janu Sirsasana* (Head to Knee Pose)
7. *Parivrtta Janu Sirsasana* (Revolved Head to Knee Pose)
8. *Ardha Matysendrasana* (Half Seated Twist Pose)
9. Repeat steps 6 through 8 on other side.

CONTINUED ON PAGE 152.

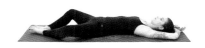

1 Supta Baddha Konasana

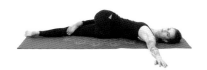

2 Supta Matsyendrasana

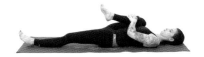

3 Supta Pavana Muktasana

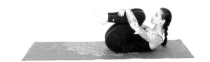

4 Apanasana

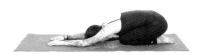

5 Balasana

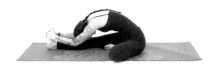

6 Janu Sirsasana

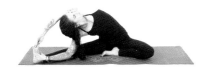

7 Parivrtta Janu Sirsasana

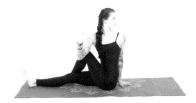

8 Ardha Matsyendrasana

151

10. *Baddha Konasana* (Seated Bound Angle Pose)

11. *Upavistha Konasana* (Seated Wide Angle Forward Bend)

12. *Gomukhasana* (Cow Face Pose). Repeat on other side.

13. *Uttanasana* (Standing Forward Fold)

14. *Anjaneyasana* (Knee Down Lunge). Repeat on other side.

15. *Adho Mukha Svanasana* (Downward Facing Dog Pose). Note: From this pose, take your feet as wide as the mat, pointing your toes out and your heels in. Slowly, start to bend your knees and walk your hands back to your feet, lifting your heels high as you do.

16. *Malasana* (Garland Pose)

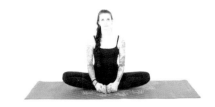

10 Baddha Konasana

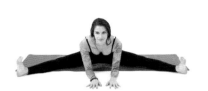

11 Upavistha Konasana

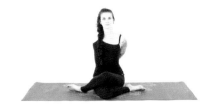

12 Gomukhasana

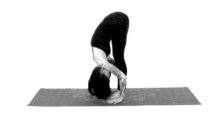

13 Uttanasana

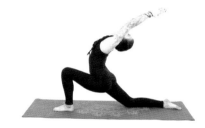

14 Anjaneyasana

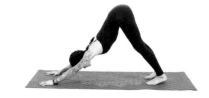

15 Adho Mukha Svanasana

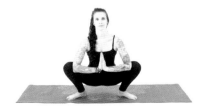

16 Malasana

Reclining Hero Pose (Supta Virasana)

My way-overused joke about Reclining Hero Pose is that it's such a deep quad stretch that you need to be a hero to get into it. In all honesty, though, if you make sure to warm up the quads and come into the pose slowly, it's not all that heroic. Have props on hand: lots of pillows and blankets. You should feel a deep stretch, but no sharp pain. Make sure you can be a hero without ripping your cape!

1. *Surya Namaskar A* (Sun Salutation A—see page 1)
2. *Natarajasana* (Dancer's Pose). Repeat other side.
3. *Utkatasana* (Chair Pose)
4. Lower to *Navasana* (Boat Pose)
5. *Purvottanasana* (Reverse Plank Pose)
6. Vinyasa to *Utkatasana* (Chair Pose)
7. Lower to *Navasana* (Boat Pose)

CONTINUED ON PAGE 156.

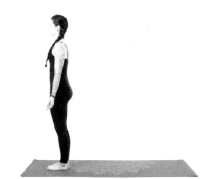

1 Sun Salutation A—
see page 1

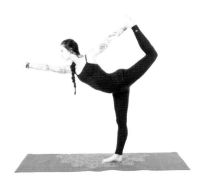

2 Natarajasana

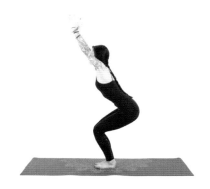

3 Utkatasana

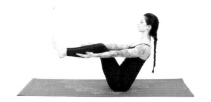

4 Navasana

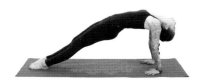

5 Purvottanasana

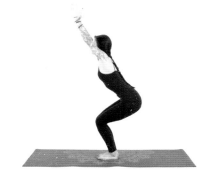

6 Utkatasana

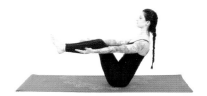

7 Navasana

8. *Ustrasana* (Camel Pose)

9. *Balasana* (Child's Pose)

10. *Bhujangasana* (Cobra Pose)

11. *Salabhasana* (Locust Pose). Repeat one time.

12. *Dhanurasana* (Bow Pose)

13. *Balasana* (Child's Pose)

14. *Baddha Konasana* (Bound Angle Pose)

Continued on page 158.

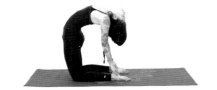

8 Ustrasana

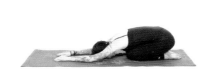

9 Balasana

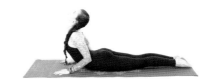

10 Bhujangasana

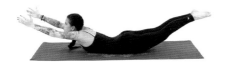

11 Salabhasana

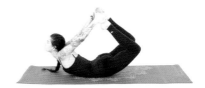

12 Dhanurasana

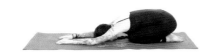

13 Balasana

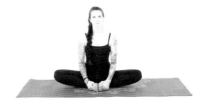

14 Baddha Konasana

15. *Upavistha Konasana* (Seated Wide Legged Forward Bend)

16. *Janu Sirsasana* (Seated Head to Knee Pose)

17. *Parivrtta Janu Sirsasana* (Revolved Head to Knee Pose)

18. Repeat steps 15 through 17 on other side.

19. *Ardha Virasana* (Half Hero's Pose). Fold forward over straightened leg before coming into the full posture. Repeat on other side.

20. *Paschimottasana* (Seated Forward Fold Pose)

21. *Virasana* (Hero Pose)

22. *Supta Virasana* (Reclining Hero Pose). Note: Recline very slowly, noticing how the knees feel in this pose. To come out of the pose, it's important to engage the navel in and up, and be aware of any sensitivity in the lower back.

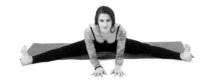

15 Upavistha Konasana

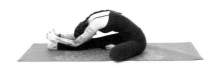

16 Janu Sirsasana

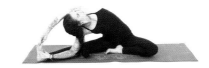

17 Parivrtta Janu Sirsasana

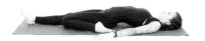

19 Ardha Virasana

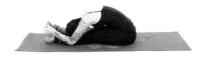

20 Paschimottanasana

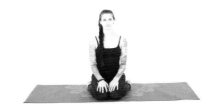

21 Virasana

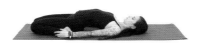

22 Supta Virasana

Resting Pigeon Pose
(Supta Eka Pada Rajakapotasana)

Resting Pigeon Pose (a variation of *Eka Pada Rajakapotasana*) is the most requested pose in the classes I teach. It's one of the hip openers that yogis either love, or love to hate. It helps stretch out the lower back and hips and also helps prepare our bodies for more intense hip openers, many of which we will play with later on in this chapter.

1. *Supta Baddha Konasana* (Reclined Bound Angle). Hold for 1–3 minutes.
2. *Ananda Balasana* (Happy Baby Pose). Note: From this pose, move into a variation of Pigeon by taking an ankle to the opposite knee and drawing both legs into the chest.
3. *Balasana* (Child's Pose)
4. Cat/Cow in Table Top. Note: Take one leg out to the side with the knee bent at a 90-degree angle, inner thigh parallel to the floor. Draw circles with the leg in both directions. Repeat on other side.
5. *Adho Mukha Svanasana* (Downward Facing Dog Pose)
6. *Vrksasana* (Tree Pose). Repeat on on other side.
7. *Garudasana* (Eagle Pose). Repeat on on other side.
8. *Uttanasana* (Standing Forward Fold)

CONTINUED ON PAGE 162.

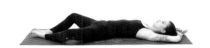

1   Supta Baddha Konasana

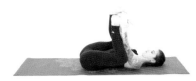

2   Ananda Balasana

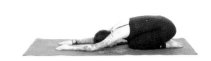

3   Balasana

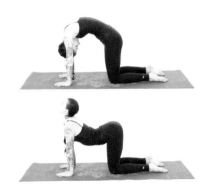

6   Cat/Cow in Table Top

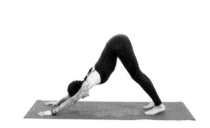

5   Adho Mukha Svanasana

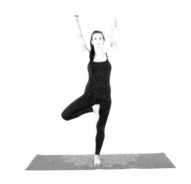

6   Vrksasana

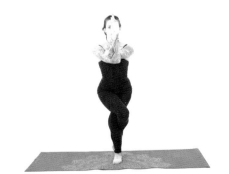

7   Garudasana

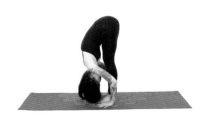

8   Uttanasana

9. *Deviasana* (Goddess Pose). Note: Take hands to the inside of the knees and roll the shoulders for an upper back opener.

10. *Ustrasana* (Camel Pose)

11. *Janu Sirsasana* (Head to Knee Pose). Repeat on other side.

12. *Baddha Konasana* (Seated Bound Angle Pose)

13. *Upavistha Konasana* (Seated Wide Angle Forward Bend)

14. *Gomukhasana* (Cow Face Pose)

15. Swing the top leg back behind you to come into *Supta Eka Pada Rajakapotasana* (Resting Pigeon Pose), readjusting the legs as needed.

16. Repeat steps 14 and 15 on other side.

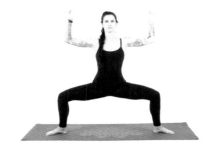

9 Deviasana

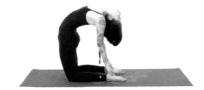

10 Ustrasana

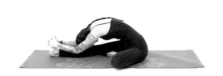

11 Janu Sirsasana

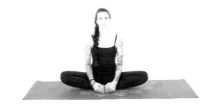

12 Baddha Konasana

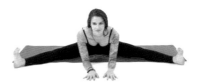

13 Upavistha Konasana

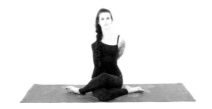

14 Gomukhasana

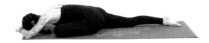

15 Supta Eka Pada
Rajakapotasana

Boat Pose (Paripurna Navasana)

Although this pose is often described as a core strengthener, the hip flexors and quads can get even more of a workout when this pose is done correctly. If your torso starts to tilt backward and your lower back rounds when you try to straighten your legs, continue to practice Boat Pose with your knees bent. Over time, and with the help of this sequence, the strength and flexibility required to practice full Boat Pose will develop.

1. *Kapalabhati Pranayama* (Skull Shining Breath) in *Virasana* (Hero Pose). Perform 1–3 rounds.

2. *Paschimottanasana* (Seated Forward Fold)

3. Cat/Cow in Table Top

4. *Adho Mukha Svanasana* (Downward Facing Dog Pose)

5. *Trikonasana* (Triangle Pose)

6. Repeat steps 4 and 5 on other side.

7. *Uttanasana* (Standing Forward Fold)

8. *Utkatasana* (Chair Pose)

9. *Utthita Hasta Padangusthasana* (Standing Hand-to-Big Toe Pose). Note: Release the hand off the foot and extend the leg, trying to keep it parallel to the earth, for 5 cycles of breath. Repeat other side.

10. *Anjaneyasana* (Knee Down Lunge)

Continued on page 166.

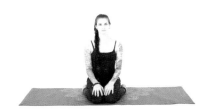

1 Virasana

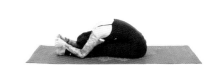

2 Paschimottanasana

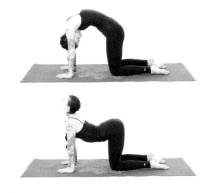

3 Cat/Cow in Table Top

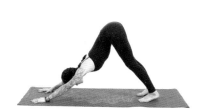

4 Adho Mukha Svanasana

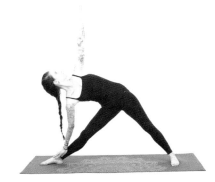

5 Trikonasana

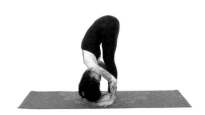

7 Uttanasana

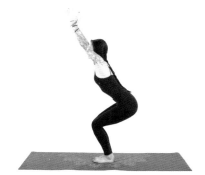

8 Utkatasana

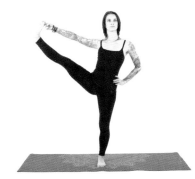

9 Utthita Hasta Padangusthasana

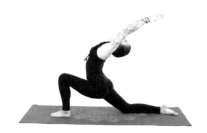

10 Anjaneyasana

11. *Ardha Hanumanasana* (Half Split Pose)

12. Flow between steps 10 and 11.

13. *Alanasana* (High Lunge Pose)

14. *Virabhadrasana III* (Warrior III Pose)

15. *Vinyasa* to repeat steps 10 through 14 on other side.

16. *Ardha Matysendrasana* (Half Seated Twist Pose). Repeat on other side.

17. *Tolasana* (Scale Pose)

18. *Navasana* (Boat Pose) Note: Practice the first round with knees bent.

19. *Baddha Konasana* (Bound Angle Pose)

20. *Paripurna Navasana* (Boat Pose)

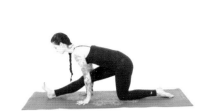

11 Ardha Hanumanasana

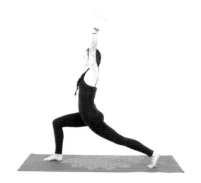

13 Alanasana

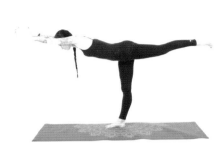

14 Virabhadrasana III

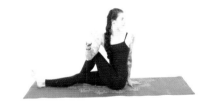

16 Ardha Matsyendrasana

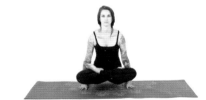

17 Tolasana

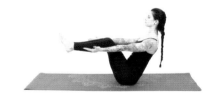

18 Navasana

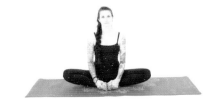

19 Baddha Konasana

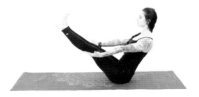

20 Navasana

Heron Pose (Krounchasana)

This pose combines the intense hamstring opening of poses like *Parsvottanasana* (Pyramid Pose) and *Utthita Hasta Padangusthasana* (Extended Hand-to-Big Toe Pose) with the quad stretch of *Ardha Virasana* (Half Hero Pose). If the quads or knees aren't up to Half Hero, keep the grounded leg bent as in *Janu Sirsasana* (Head to Knee Pose) or *Vrksasana* (Tree Pose).

1. *Supta Padangusthasana* (Reclined Big Toe Pose)
2. *Supta Trivikramasana* (Reclined Vishnu Pose)
3. *Urdhva Mukha Paschimottanasana* (Upward Facing Forward Fold Pose)
4. Repeat steps 1 through 3 on other side.
5. *Dandasana* (Staff Pose)
6. *Paschimottanasana* (Seated Forward Fold)
7. *Baddha Konasana* (Bound Angle Pose)
8. *Janu Sirsasana* (Head to Knee Pose). Repeat on other side.
9. *Anjaneyasana* (Knee Down Lunge)
10. *Ardha Hanumanasana* (Half Split Pose)
11. Flow between steps 9 and 10.
12. *Parsvotttanasana* (Pyramid Pose)
13. Repeat steps 9 through 12 on other side.
14. *Adho Mukha Svanasana* (Downward Facing Dog Pose)

Continued on page 170.

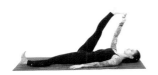

1 Supta
Padangusthasana

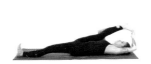

2 Supta
Trivikramasana

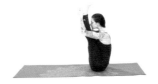

3 Urdhva Mukha
Paschimottanasana

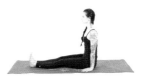

5 Dandasana

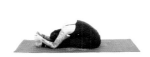

6 Paschimottanasana

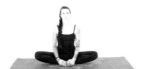

7 Baddha Konasana

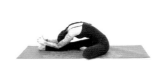

8 Janu Sirsasana

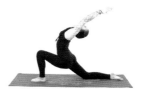

9 Anjaneyasana

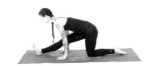

10 Ardha
Hanumanasana

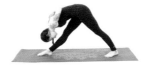

12 Parsvottanasana

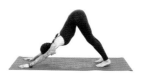

14 Adho Mukha
Svanasana

15. *Uttanasana* (Standing Forward Fold)

16. *Urdhva Hastasana* (Upward Hands Pose). Note: Add lots of yummy side stretches!

17. *Utkatasana* (Chair Pose)

18. *Natarajasana* (Dancer's Pose). Repeat other side.

19. *Utkatasana* (Chair Pose)

20. Lower to *Navasana* (Boat Pose)

21. *Purvottanasana* (Reverse Plank Pose)

22. *Ardha Virasana* (Half Hero's Pose). Fold forward over straightened leg before coming into the full posture. Repeat on other side with a *Vinyasa* after each side.

23. *Paschimottasana* (Seated Forward Fold Pose)

24. *Virasana* (Hero Pose)

25. *Krounchasana* (Heron Pose). Repeat on other side.

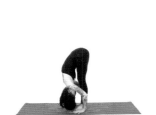

15 Uttanasana

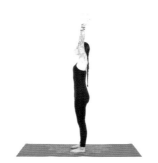

16 Urdhva Hastasana

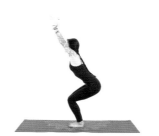

17 Utkatasana

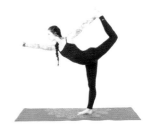

18 Natarajasana

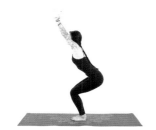

19 Utkatasana

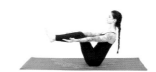

20 Navasana

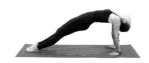

21 Purvottanasana

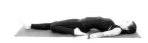

22 Ardha Virasana

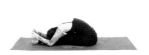

23 Paschimottanasana

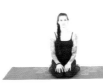

24 Virasana

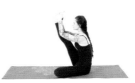

25 Krounchasana

Firelog Pose (Agnistambhasana)

This pose is sometimes called Double Pigeon, because, essentially, that's what's going on here. Take whatever hip openness and flexibility you gain in Resting Pigeon Pose and multiply by two. Not so bad, right?

1. *Supta Baddha Konasana* (Reclined Bound Angle Pose)
2. *Supta Matsyendrasana* (Supine Twist). Note: After this pose, move into a variation of Pigeon by taking an ankle to the opposite knee and drawing both legs into the chest.
3. Repeat step 2 on other side.
4. *Ananda Balasana* (Happy Baby Pose)
5. *Paschimottanasana* (Seated Forward Fold)
6. Cat/Cow in Table Top
7. *Adho Mukha Svanasana* (Downward Facing Dog Pose)
8. *Uttanasana* (Standing Forward Fold). Note: Take hands to opposite elbow for Rag Doll.
9. *Vrksasana* (Tree Pose). Note: As in step 2, take the ankle above the opposite knee. Bend the knee and fold forward, bringing hands to bricks or the ground. Repeat on other side.

Continued on page 174.

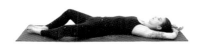

1 Supta Baddha Konasana

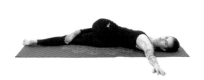

2 Supta Matsyendrasana

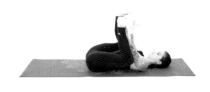

4 Ananda Balasana

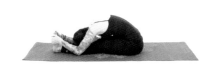

5 Paschimottanasana

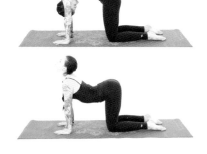

6 Cat/Cow in Table Top

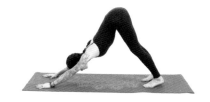

7 Adho Mukha Svanasana

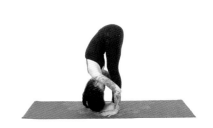

8 Uttanasana

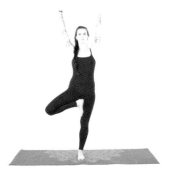

9 Vrksasana

10. *Malasana* (Garland Pose)

11. *Janu Sirsasana* (Head to Knee Pose). Repeat on other side.

12. *Baddha Konasana* (Seated Bound Angle Pose)

13. *Upavistha Konasana* (Seated Wide Angle Forward Fold)

14. *Gomukhasana* (Cow Face Pose). Repeat other side.

15. *Supta Eka Pada Rajakapotasana* (Resting Pigeon Pose)

16. *Agnistambhasana* (Firelog Pose)

17. Repeat steps 15 and 16 on other side.

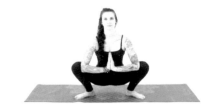

10 Malasana

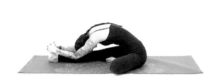

11 Janu Sirsasana

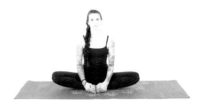

12 Baddha Konasana

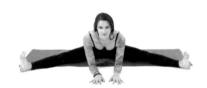

13 Upavistha Konasana

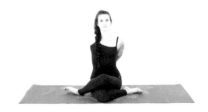

14 Gomukhasana

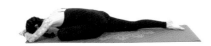

15 Supta Eka Pada Rajakapotasana

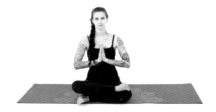

16 Agnistambhasana

Tortoise Pose (Kurmasana)

Allow your attention to draw inward just like a turtle draws into its shell while you are in Tortoise Pose. Notice the fluctuations of the breath and the wandering of the mind while experiencing a deep forward fold and hamstring stretch.

1. *Tadasana* (Mountain Pose)

2. *Surya Namaskar A* (Sun Salutation A—see page 1). Repeat 5 times.

3. *Garudasana* (Eagle Pose). Repeat on other side.

4. *Uttanasana* (Standing Forward Fold). Hold for 1–2 minutes.

5. *Utkatasana* (Chair Pose)

6. *Parivrtta Utkatasana* (Revolved Chair Pose). Repeat on other side.

7. *Prasarita Padottanasana* (Standing Wide-Legged Forward Fold)

8. *Prasarita Padottanasana* (Standing Wide-Legged Forward Fold), with *Gomukhasana* (Cow Face Pose) bind in the arms. Repeat with other arm on top.

9. *Adho Mukha Svanasana* (Downward Facing Dog Pose). Note: Pedal the heels in place.

10. *Virabhadrasana II* (Warrior II)

Continued on page 178.

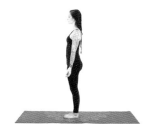

1 Tadasana

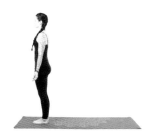

2 Sun Salutation A— see page 1

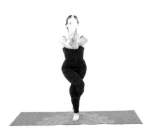

3 Garudasana

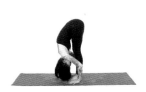

4 Uttanasana

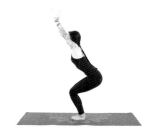

5 Utkatasana

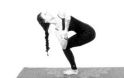

6 Parivrtta Utkatasana

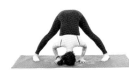

7 Prasarita Padottanasana

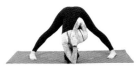

8 Prasarita Padottanasana with Gomukhasana

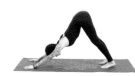

9 Adho Mukha Svanasana

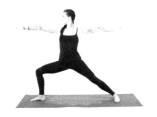

10 Virabhadrasana II

11. *Trikonasana* (Triangle Pose)

12. *Baddha Utthita Parsvakonasana* (Bound Extended Side Angle Pose)

13. *Vinyasa* to repeat steps 9 through 12 on other side.

14. *Malasana* (Garland Pose)

15. *Paschimottanasana* (Seated Forward Fold)

16. *Purvottanasana* (Reverse Plank Pose)

17. *Ardha Virasana* (Half Hero's Pose). Fold forward over straightened leg before coming into the full posture.

18. *Baddha Konasana* (Bound Angle Pose)

19. *Upavistha Konasana* (Seated Wide Angle Forward Bend)

20. *Kurmasana* (Tortoise Pose)

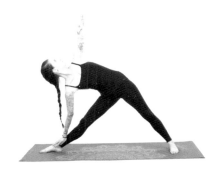

11 Trikonasana

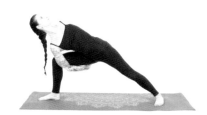

12 Baddha Utthita
Parsvakonasana

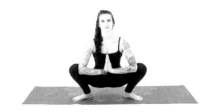

14 Malasana

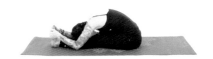

15 Paschimottanasana

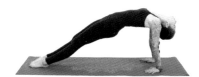

16 Purvottanasana

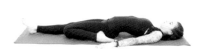

17 Ardha Virasana

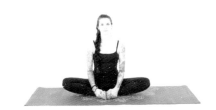

18 Baddha Konasana

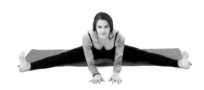

19 Upavistha Konasana

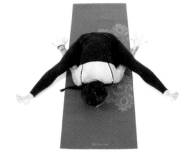

20 Kurmasana

Frog Pose (Mandukasana Frog Pose)

Not to be confused with *Bhekasana*, also translated as Frog Pose (perhaps there were many types of frogs back in the days of naming extremely challenging yoga poses). In this variation of Frog, get ready for the hip opener of your life. Deepen the stretch by taking the knees wider apart or gently pressing the hips toward the heels.

1. *Supta Baddha Konasana* (Reclined Bound Angle Pose)

2. *Ananda Balasana* (Happy Baby Pose)

3. Cat/Cow in Table. Note: Take one leg out to the side at a 90-degree angle to the floor. Draw circles with leg in both directions. Repeat on other side.

4. Sphinx Pose. Note: Focus on drawing the core in and lengthening the spine. Use this action in Frog Pose, as well.

5. *Adho Mukha Svanasana* (Downward Facing Dog Pose)

6. *Tadasana* (Mountain Pose)

7. *Vrkasana* (Tree Pose). Repeat on other side.

Continued on page 182.

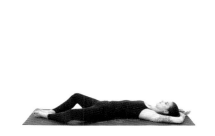

1 Supta Baddha Konasana

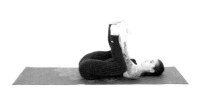

2 Ananda Balasana

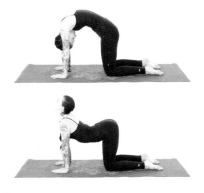

3 Cat/Cow in Table Top

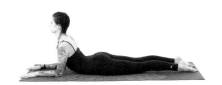

4 Sphinx

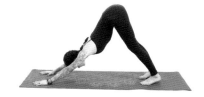

5 Adho Mukha Svanasana

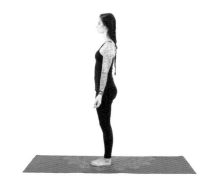

6 Tadasana

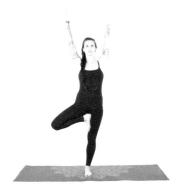

7 Vrksasana

8. *UTKATASANA* (Chair Pose)

9. *MALASANA* (Garland Pose)

10. *UTTANASANA* (Standing Forward Fold)

11. Flow between steps 9 and 10 with the breath, ending in a forward fold.

12. *VIRABHADRASANA II* (Warrior II)

13. *DEVIASANA* (Goddess Pose). Note: Hold this pose for 5 cycles of breath, bending and straightening the knees with the breath.

14. Repeat steps 12 and 13 on other side.

15. *JANU SIRSASANA* (Head to Knee Pose). Repeat on other side.

16. *MANDUKASANA* (Frog Pose)

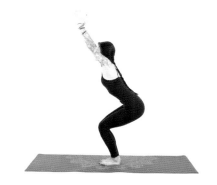

8 Utkatasana

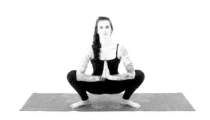

9 Malasana

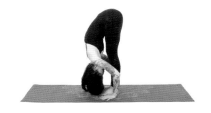

10 Uttanasana

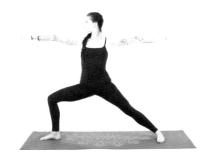

12 Virabhadrasana II

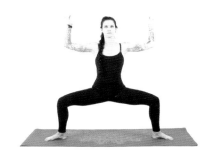

13 Deviasana

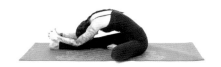

15 Janu Sirsasana

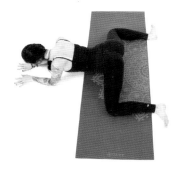

16 Mandukasana

Full Splits (Hanumanasana)

When coming out of this pose, I often see students torqueing their front leg from side to side so they don't curl up their mat. Please don't do this; I'd rather your mat get all crunched up than your knee. Blocks can be useful underneath the hands as well as underneath the front thigh and the back quad while you are gaining flexibility.

1. *SUPTA VIRASANA* (Reclined Hero Pose). Note: Come into the restorative version of this pose, using as many pillows as you like behind the back.
2. *SUPTA BADDHA KONASANA* (Reclined Bound Angle Pose)
3. *ANANDA BALASANA* (Happy Baby Pose)
4. *SUPTA PADANGUSTHASANA* (Reclined Big Toe Pose)
5. *SUPTA TRIVIKRAMASANA* (Reclined Vishnu Pose)
6. *SUPTA PARIVRTTA PADANGUSTHASANA* (Reclining Revolved Hand-to-Big Toe Pose**)**
7. Repeat steps 3 through 6 on other side.
8. Cat/Cow in Table Top
9. *ADHO MUKHA SVANASANA* (Downward Facing Dog Pose)
10. *ANJANEYASANA* (Knee Down Lunge)
11. *ARDHA HANUMANASANA* (Half Split Pose)
12. Flow between steps 10 and 11 as many times as you like. Repeat on other side.
13. *SURYA NAMASKAR B* (Sun Salutation B—see page 2). Repeat 5 times, substituting *ALANASANA* (High Lunge Pose) for *VIRABHADRASANA I* (Warrior I Pose) in the sequence.

CONTINUED ON PAGE 186.

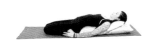

1 Supta Virasana

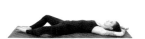

2 Supta Baddha Konasana

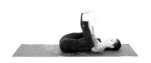

3 Ananda Balasana

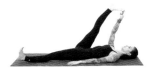

4 Supta Padangusthasana

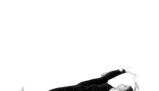

5 Supta Trivikramasana

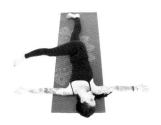

6 Supta Parivrtta Padangusthasana

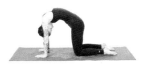

8 Cat/Cow in Table Top

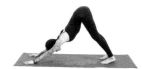

9 Adho Mukha Svanasana

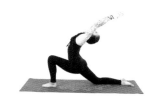

10 Anjaneyasana

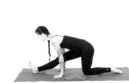

11 Ardha Hanumanasana

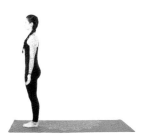

13 Sun Salutation B—see page 2

14. *Uttanasana* (Standing Forward Fold)

15. *Adho Mukha Svanasana* (Downward Facing Dog)

16. *Trikonasana* (Triangle Pose)

17. *Ardha Chandrasana* (Balancing Half Moon Pose)

18. *Natarajasana* (Dancer's Pose)

19. *Urdhva Prasarita Eka Padasana* (Standing Splits)

20. *Parsvottanasana* (Pyramid Pose)

21. *Utthan Pristhasana* (Lizard Pose)

22. *Supta Eka Pada Rajakapotasana* (Resting Pigeon Pose)

23. *Adho Mukha Svanasana* (Downward Facing Dog)

24. *Hanumanasana* (Splits)

25. Repeat steps 14 through 24 on other side.

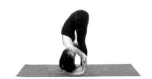

14 Uttanasana

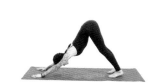

15 Adho Mukha
Svanasana

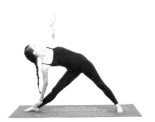

16 Trikonasana

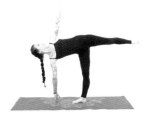

17 Ardha
Chandrasana

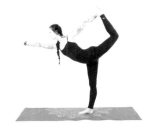

18 Natarajasana

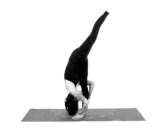

19 Urdhva Prasarita
Eka Padasana

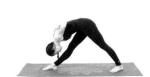

20 Parsvottanasana

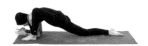

21 Utthan Pristhasana

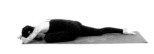

22 Supta Eka Pada
Rajakapotasana

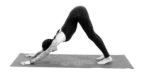

23 Adho Mukha Svanasana

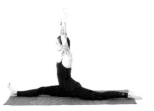

24 Hanumanasana

Lotus Pose (*Padmasana*)

Lotus Pose is mentioned in the earliest texts on classical hatha yoga. This venerable posture is used for meditation, *Pranayama*, and its many physical benefits. It's said that wherever the Buddha walked, lotus flowers bloomed. These days, however, the Dalai Lama advises using a cushion, blanket, or some other support underneath your seat while practicing the pose. Here, I will suggest the same.

1. *Janu Sirsasana* (Head to Knee Pose)
2. *Parivrtta Janu Sirsasana* (Revolved Head to Knee Pose)
3. *Upavistha Konasana* (Seated Wide Angle Forward Bend)
4. Repeat steps 1 through 3 on other side.
5. *Baddha Konasana* (Bound Angle Pose)
6. *Surya Namaskar A* (Sun Salutation A—see page 1). Repeat 5 times.
7. *Surya Namaskar B* (Sun Salutation B—see page 2). Repeat 5 times.
8. *Deviasana* (Goddess Pose)
9. *Prasarita Padottanasana* (Standing Wide-Legged Forward Fold)
10. *Utthita Pavana Muktasana* (Standing Wind Relieving Pose). Repeat other side.
11. *Natarajasana* (Dancer's Pose). Repeat other side.
12. *Ardha Baddha Padmottanasana* (Half Bound Standing Lotus Forward Fold). Repeat other side.

Continued on page 190.

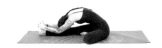

1 Janu Sirsasana

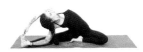

2 Parivrtta Janu Sirsasana

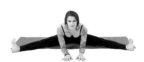

3 Upavistha Konasana

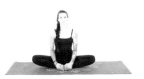

5 Baddha Konasana

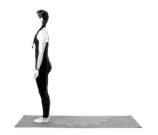

6 Sun Salutation A— see page 1

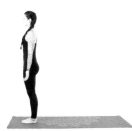

7 Sun Salutation B—see page 2

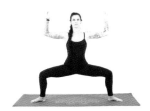

8 Deviasana

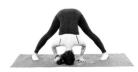

9 Prasarita Padottanasana

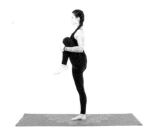

10 Utthita Pavana Muktasana

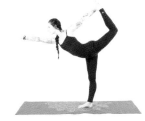

11 Natarajasana

12 Ardha Baddha Padmottanasana

13. Cat/Cow in Table Top

14. *Ardha Virasana* (Half Hero Pose). Repeat on other side.

15. *Ardha Matsyendrasana* (Half Seated Twist). Repeat on other side.

16. *Paschimottanasana* (Seated Forward Fold)

17. *Supta Eka Pada Rajakapotasana* (Resting Pigeon Pose). Repeat on other side.

18. *Ustrasana* (Camel Pose)

19. *Balasana* (Child's Pose)

20. *Padmasana* (Lotus Pose)

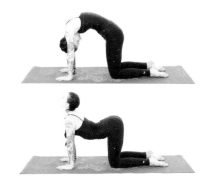

13 Cat/Cow in Table Top

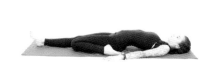

14 Ardha Virasana

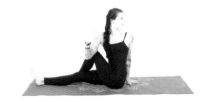

15 Ardha Matsyendrasana

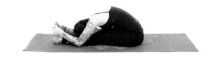

16 Paschimottanasana

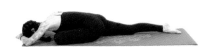

17 Supta Eka Pada
Rajakapotasana

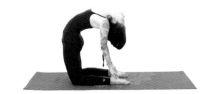

18 Ustrasana

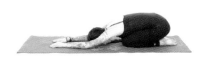

19 Balasana

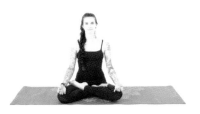

20 Padmasana

Cool Down

A Restorative Sequence and Savasana

Bonus: A Restorative Closing Sequence

1. *BALASANA* (Child's Pose). Note: "Thread the needle" in Child's Pose, taking one arm underneath the other to rest on the shoulder and upper arm. Repeat on other side.

2. *ANANDA BALASANA* (Happy Baby Pose)

3. *SUPTA BADDHA KONASANA* (Reclined Bound Angle Pose)

4. *SUPTA MATSYENDRASANA* (Supine Twist Pose). Repeat on other side.

5. *VIPARITA KARANI* (Legs Up the Wall Pose). Note: Take one ankle across the opposite thigh above the knee ("Ankle to Knee" Pose). Repeat on other side.

6. *SAVASANA* (Corpse Pose)

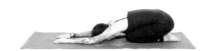

1   Balasana

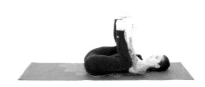

2   Ananda Balasana

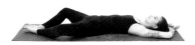

3   Supta Baddha Konasana

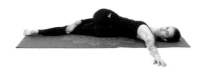

4   Supta Matsyendrasana

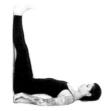

5   Viparita Karani

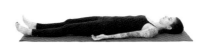

6   Savasana

Acknowledgments

Those who know me well know that I'm a mediocre cook at best, but a very appreciative eater. At the book launch party for my first book, *The Joy of Yoga,* I took some time to give thanks to those who fed me—spiritually and emotionally, sure, but mostly those who stood in their kitchen and made me a meal. In writing *Yoga Twists and Turns,* the following people kept me in good health, spirits, and caloric intake: Rachel VerValin (in-between class snacks), Steph Green (kimchi pancakes), Linden McBride (Dutch pancakes), Caitlin Schickel (Italian), Anaar D-S and Ethan Winn (Indian; birthday cake), Anna Angel (basically the same things I cook), Laurel Stewart (pawpaw ice cream), Erin Camp and Yamin Chevellard (tea; chocolate), Chelsea Morris (popovers), Dara Silverman (seder), Brad DeFrees (Viva), Emma Frisch (pickled deliciousness), Elizabeth Herendeen (salmon), Jenna A-D and Ari R-M (mushrooms), Hayden and Ro Kantor (Indian), Sarah Kelsen (ramps), Megan Shehan and Graham Rowlands (salad party; everything), Shoshi Perrey (inspired cocktails), Katie Stoner (homemade pasta), and Hannah Volpi (dates, figs). An extra special shout-out goes to Christina Black, who fed me at least once or twice a week, and came up with my tagline: "Emma Silverman: the only yoga teacher who's never bullsh*tted me."

After I finished the rough draft of this book, I sent out a copy to a group of amazing yoga teachers, yogis, and writers. Jenni C-R not only gave notes, but scanned and emailed them to me. Zainab Zakari engaged with me in an epic back-and-forth about the correct Sanksrit term for Pigeon Pose (I'm still not sure I got it right) and was meticulous in her edits. Ilana Berman and Nicole Stumpf gave it a read, and basically just told me that they loved me and everything was perfect, which is exactly what I needed during that hectic time. Megan Shehan edited the document so thoroughly, and responded to me so quickly with her suggestions, that I had to re-send out the document to everyone else letting them know that a few (thousand) mistakes were already caught. And, of course, there's Yardenne Greenspan. I tricked Yardenne into being my friend by promising her we could have work dates, and then never shut up when we got together. I am so glad we never got any work done.

To my editor, Nicole Frail: As always, it was a pleasure. Clarity is the thing I value most in communication with others, and Nicole is the ideal.

To my fairy godmother, Kathleen Rushall: Ultimately, the reason any of this happened.

To my teachers: to Ilana Berman for being my sister, to Nicole Stumpf for being my twin, and to both for being true soul-friends. And to Elizabeth Gabriel for teaching grace by example.

To tiny babies: Asa, August, Ayla, Charlotte, Eliana, Laya, and Orion; with gratitude to their parents.

To my bosses: Heather Healey at Mighty Yoga, Tory Jenis at Blackbird Yoga and Pilates, and Emily Ellison and Diane Fine at Cornell University.

To my best men: Sam Whitehead and Ben Savitzky.

To my Rockers: Erica Webb, Heather Fisch, Saro Hinson, and Ruth Ballenzweig.

To my oldest, best friend: Sara Giffin.

And to my family: I figured I would never, ever be allowed to write a second book, so I dedicated the first one to everyone instead of giving each their own book. The truth is, everything is dedicated to my family—past, present, future, every step of the way. So this is for them, too. And this. And this.

Thank you for everything. I have no complaints whatsoever.